Real-Life Detox

By Chet Zelasko, Ph.D.

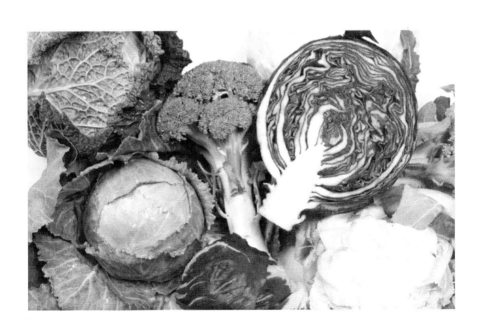

Published by Zelasko Media

Chet Zelasko PhD LLC
POB 888633
Grand Rapids, MI 49588
Website: www.drchet.com

The health information in this book is designed for educational purposes only. It's not a substitute for medical advice from your healthcare provider, and you should not use it to diagnose or treat a health problem or disease. It's designed to motivate you to work toward better health, and that includes seeing your healthcare professional regularly. If what you've read raises any questions or concerns about health problems or possible diseases, talk to your healthcare provider today.

Table of Contents

Part One:

How to Cleanse and Detox

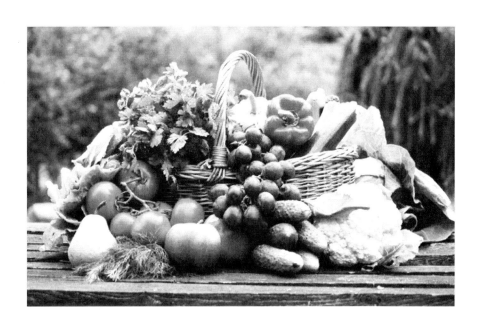

Why You Need This Book

Real-Life Detox is designed to help you feel better, have more energy, and reduce your risk of serious disease, depending on how you integrate the information into your everyday life. I'll also give you the science behind it in a way that's easy to understand. I'm going to tell you what's real and what's not when it comes to detoxifying your body.

Let's face it: there's a lot of confusion about detoxification programs. Some use a crazy concoction of foods, spices, and herbs; most that I've seen confuse a digestive cleansing program with a detoxification program. While the two may seem to be related and the process may seem similar, they're two different things.

And then there are the healthcare professionals. They're firmly entrenched in science-based medicine and can't understand why we would need to do anything extra to accomplish what the body is supposed to do anyway. They read about the lemon juice, maple syrup, and cayenne pepper "cleanse" and think that's what detoxification is all about. And yet, they have to know that the detoxification process that takes place in the body is legitimate: it uses the same systems that the body uses to eliminate pharmaceuticals when they're done working in our bodies. Whether that detoxification system works well is the question they don't seem willing to acknowledge.

Speaking of the detoxification process, I'm going to explain how that works. In the process, I'll answer many questions about detoxification. Let me give you a few:

- Can you really help your digestive system stop the bloating and overall lousiness you feel?

- Are there special nutrients that you need during a detox program?
- Can herbs really help with the detoxification process? What does the science show?
- What nutrients can you eat every day to help regularly detoxify your body?
- Can you reduce the risk of diseases by eating a better diet—not for just a day, three days, or a week, but for the rest of your life?

That's a pretty ambitious list, but that's what I'm going to cover in this book.

When I gave this book the title *Real-Life Detox*, I wanted you to understand that this book will be easy to read, easy to follow, and easy to incorporate into your real life. The goal is to help you feel better, have more energy, and maybe, have fewer health issues—all while keeping your real life moving forward.

We have a tendency to try to fix things, especially our bodies, in a short period of time. I'm sorry, but that's just not possible in most cases, and that includes detoxifying our bodies. I believe adding small changes to your lifestyle on a regular basis is the most effective way to help you get and stay healthy. However, that doesn't mean that you can't do something slightly dramatic, let's say over a weekend, that can help get you pointed in the right direction.

If you're familiar with the now-retired comic strip "Cathy," there was a significant strip on New Year's Day many years ago. It went something like this: Cathy had set New Year's resolutions to eat better, lose weight, and exercise. When she woke up New Year's Day, she ate a donut. Well, that blew her diet for the day. Because the day was shot, the week was shot. And because she blew the week, the month was blown. And because the month was gone, she had messed up the entire year. Game over.

That's the way too many of us approach how we treat our bodies, but when it comes to detoxifying your body, there's no all in or all out. I believe you can make small changes that will have a profound effect on your body:

- You can have more energy.
- Your digestive system can feel better.
- You can optimize your detoxification system.

Not by drinking lemon juice with maple syrup and cayenne pepper, sitting in a sweat lodge, or eating half your lawn, but by making small changes in what you eat and making those changes a regular part of your lifestyle. That's what *Real-Life Detox* is all about.

How to Use This Book

I've thought a long time about the organization of this book. If you read my weekly messages or have attended one of my seminars, you know I'm always concerned with why: Why detox? Why cleanse? Why try to eliminate problem foods from your diet? On and on. I realized a little while ago that might not be the most important thing to some of you—you may just want to know what to do and how to do it, so that's the way the book is organized: Part One is *what* and *how to*, and Part Two is *why*.

In Part One, each chapter will give you a summary of the concept; then I'll explain what to do and how to do it. I'll also explain the elements of other cleansing and detox programs that aren't really necessary.

When we're done with the *what* and the *how*, I'll give you the *why* for each part as supported by the benefits to your health and the science in Part Two, but you really need to know only what and how—you can skip the why for now and get on with your detox. But the science is really fascinating, so I hope you'll check out Part Two as well.

Part Three contains the recipes you'll use in the detox program and later in your daily life to keep your detoxification system working effectively.

I'm approaching this process in a straightforward and simple way: food first, nutrients in supplement form second, and if the science warrants it, herbs as well. Those are my priorities in putting together this practical and easy-to-use book.

The Difference Between a Cleanse and Detox

The first order of business is to clearly define what we mean by a detoxification program. People use the expression "I'm going to do a cleanse" or "I'm going to do a detox" interchangeably; the problem is that they're not the same process, although they may involve similar procedures such as modifying what you eat and drink. The main difference is that they do not focus on the same organs:

- The digestive system, which would be the focus of a cleanse, is related to the breakdown of food, absorption of nutrients, and elimination of waste products.
- The liver is the detoxification organ; its job is to pull all the toxins from your bloodstream.

While they're intimately related in working together and the digestive system is certainly involved in detoxification by eliminating waste, they're two different processes, and each can cause problems by itself. You can have problems with chronic constipation and yet have no real issues with detoxification. Or you may feel lethargic and fatigued because of the inability of your liver to eliminate toxins and yet have no issues with your gut.

Getting your digestive system to operate at peak efficiency and your liver performing its detoxification function regularly are clearly both important. Some of the same actions, such as drinking more water, may benefit both. But they're different because, as I said earlier, they involve different organs. With that in mind, let's begin by defining our terms as used in this book.

Cleanse

I know from the questions I get on a regular basis that many people are troubled by digestive issues—constipation, diarrhea, acid reflux, or gluten intolerance. Even more serious are ulcers, irritable bowel syndrome, and Crohn's disease. One approach to dealing with both simple and complex digestive issues is to clean out the digestive system periodically and start over.

One of the best reasons to do a cleansing program is that it utilizes a process that our ancestors were forced to endure on a regular basis: fasting. Not planned fasts for religious reasons—what I mean is the feast and famine that every culture had to endure when food was abundant during times of good crops or when food was scarce. Fasting wasn't by choice; fasting was the result of literally not having enough food, and our bodies adapted. Once modern refrigeration and transportation were developed, that changed. In modern society, food shortages don't happen very often so we eat every day; in less developed regions of the world, fasting that leads to starvation is still a significant issue.

Here's our working definition of a cleanse:

> **Cleansing means a controlled fast with the objective of cleaning out the digestive system and restoring it to normal function.**

The simplest way to cleanse is to avoid all food and just drink fluids. That can be stressful for any person who has a metabolic problem such as pre-diabetes. In addition to that, while drinking only liquids can empty the digestive system, it doesn't help it work more effectively. There's more we can do to help our gut return to optimal functioning.

Detox

When most people hear the word detoxification, they think of someone trying to quit drug or alcohol addiction. That word association is changing as the concept of detoxing the body from everyday exposure to chemicals and toxins becomes more mainstream. It's important to start with a clear definition:

> **Detoxification is the process of refreshing and restoring the biochemical systems in the body that eliminate natural and man-made toxins.**

Eliminating toxic substances can help us feel better and improve our health. How do you enhance that system? By eating specific vegetables and fruits that contain the nutrients that the detoxification system in your body needs for optimal function. There are nutrients found in supplements that are also beneficial.

Now that we understand the difference between a cleanse and a detox, let's move on to how to accomplish both while living your real life.

The Cleanse

Cleansing Nutrition

The key to any cleanse is to minimally impact the fluid balance in the body while providing nutrients that can eliminate any remaining remnants of food; in other words, choosing nutrients that have a laxative effect along with nutrients that can begin to restore the natural intestinal bacteria.

Water
Drinking water is a fundamental part of the cleanse. In addition, the type of water you drink is important; it should be purified to eliminate contaminants and naturally occurring organisms such as bacteria. Distilled water is acceptable, but distillation eliminates the minerals; drinking too much distilled water can dilute the body's electrolytes.

Lemon and Lime
Use these liberally to add flavor to the water. You can squeeze fresh lemons and limes yourself or you can buy lemon or lime juice—whatever is more convenient for your lifestyle.

Herbal Tea
There are many varieties of herbal tea, but the two that are particularly good for the digestive system are chamomile tea and ginger tea. The tea can be drunk warm or cold with a twist of lemon. If you want to use a sweetener, let's keep it natural for now: use locally-sourced honey or one of the many stevia products on the market.

Green Tea
Green tea contains phytochemicals that are beneficial for the entire body. If you can purchase whole-leaf green tea and brew it yourself, that's the best option. There are many types of

green tea available today from online stores dedicated to selling leaf tea as well as local stores where you can sample before you buy. If that's not possible, using green tea in bags is convenient. If you're reducing your caffeine intake, use only water-processed decaffeinated green tea during the cleanse and detox.

Hot or cold doesn't matter, but keep the fluids flowing into your body regularly. For example, you can use hot green tea in the morning and then switch to iced green tea in the afternoon. If you're not crazy about the taste of green tea, you can combine it with herbal tea or even everyday tea for a different flavor; use decaf versions if that's what you prefer but it's not necessary.

Supplements

Probiotic with FOS
These are the beneficial bacteria that should be found in your digestive system. Use a probiotic with at least one billion live cultures and many varieties of bacteria. It should also include FOS, which stands for fructooligosaccharides, a sugar found in fruit. Because you won't be eating during the cleansing program, it's important to use a probiotic that contains this sugar to help the bacteria grow and thrive.

Multivitamin-Multimineral
Look for one with plant concentrates, a great source of phytonutrients. The supplement should contain at least the Recommended Dietary Allowance (RDA) of vitamins and minerals and include the primary antioxidants: vitamins C and E and the mineral selenium.

Fiber

Fiber can have a laxative effect and will help prevent constipation during the cleansing process; the goal is to get at least 15 to 25 grams of fiber per day during the cleansing program. Insoluble fiber such as psyllium adds bulk to the stool by absorbing water, but can be gritty; psyllium fiber has recently been manufactured in a form that has been ground finer to avoid the gritty feel. One thing to remember is that you shouldn't let insoluble fiber sit for any length of time—it will absorb liquid and turn into a slimy gel that you probably won't want to swallow. When I told someone how to make the Fiber Cocktail, he put it into a blender and blended it together then left for a few minutes. When he got back, he was dealing with a solid instead of a liquid. He couldn't get it down and thought I was joking. So don't mix it until you're ready to drink it! Soluble fiber such as inulin, dextrin, guar gum, and pectin mix completely in water; they have no taste and most will not thicken drinks.

Fiber Cocktail

1 teaspoon soluble fiber
1 teaspoon insoluble fiber
1 dose probiotic
8 ounces water

Mix until everything is dissolved or mostly dissolved and drink, then follow with another 8 ounces water. Soluble fiber is generally 5 grams per teaspoon while insoluble fiber is about 3 grams per teaspoon.

I do this once a day every day and three times a day when doing the cleanse. Along with the fiber, make sure to keep drinking fluids to reduce the potential for constipation.

Digestive Enzymes

These can help if you're going to use protein drinks in your cleanse. The digestive-enzyme supplement you use should contain a protease or peptidase to digest protein, a lipase to digest fat, various amylases and carboxylases to digest carbohydrates, and a lactase to digest milk products.

Magnesium
If you have a problem with chronic constipation, add magnesium—it has a slight laxative effect for most people. Take 150 mg three times per day for the two days. Magnesium is usually combined with calcium and vitamin D, both of which are acceptable during the cleansing program.

Choosing the Right Cleansing Program

The goal of the cleansing programs is to reduce food intake, clean out the digestive system, and begin the restoration of beneficial bacteria.

This book has three approaches to a cleansing program, each lasting two days. If you want to continue longer, that's okay, but I've designed the programs to be convenient and most people have two days off work every week. I'd definitely recommend a weekend because experience has shown me that a cleanse will affect your bathroom habits.

You're going to focus on sustaining fluid levels and not eating solid food of any kind. The difference between the approaches is whether or not you're getting any calories—some people just can't make it two days without calories and that's okay; you know your body best and what it needs. I've designed the Cleansing Program so that just about anyone can do at least one approach. If you start with Cleanse 1 or 2 and find you don't have enough energy to do what you have to do, move up a level.

Cleanse 1: Almost No Calories

This approach will work best over a weekend or for those with relatively sedentary jobs, rather than jobs that involve strenuous physical labor.

Cleanse 2: Limited Calories

This approach will work best for those who need to sustain their energy levels because of work or play. The calories come from vegetable and fruit juice—fresh squeezed is best but not always possible. Vegetable and fruit juices can be used just as you find them in the store, but remember that fruit juice has more calories than vegetable juices normally have, so use them sparingly.

Cleanse 3: Moderate Calories

This approach works best for people with strenuous jobs who need more calories to sustain their energy levels throughout the day. It's also appropriate for people with diabetes (with their doctor's permission) or hypoglycemia. The goal is to get about 100 to 150 calories every couple of hours in a drink that's high in protein, moderate in carbohydrates, and low in fat. You can use one of the protein drink recipes in the Recipes section or buy a protein drink. Rice or vegetable protein is the best source during the program, but if you have no problem digesting soy or whey protein, those are acceptable as well.

Cleanse 1: Almost No Calories

Drink Schedule

Water, water with lemon or lime, green tea, and herbal teas:

- Immediately after waking, drink one cup of water with lemon or lime.
- Then drink one or two cups of the above fluids every waking hour.

Supplements

Probiotic	Morning and evening
Magnesium	150 mg morning, noon, and evening
Multivitamin-Multimineral	As directed on the label
Omega-3 Fatty Acids	3 grams of fish oil, flaxseed oil, or a combination
Fiber	Soluble and insoluble fiber added to drinks 2 to 4 times per day

Remember that you're not eating any food, so adding fiber is important; the goal is 15 to 25 grams per day.

Cleanse 2: Limited Calories

Drink Schedule

Water, water with lemon or lime, green tea, and herbal teas:

- Immediately after waking, drink one cup of water with lemon or lime.
- Then drink one or two cups of the above fluids every waking hour.

Vegetable juice or diluted fruit juice:

- Drink one cup an hour after rising, then every two hours as needed.

Supplements

Probiotic	Morning and evening
Magnesium	150 mg morning, noon, and evening
Multivitamin-Multimineral	As directed on the label
Omega-3 Fatty Acids	3 grams of fish oil, flaxseed oil, or a combination
Fiber	Soluble fiber and insoluble added to drinks 2 to 4 times per day

The amount of fiber added depends on the amount of fiber in the juice and whether it has fiber added; the goal is 15 to 25 grams.

Cleanse 3: Moderate Calories

Drink Schedule

Water, water with lemon or lime, green tea, and herbal teas:

- Immediately after waking, drink one cup of water with lemon or lime.
- Then drink one or two cups of the above fluids every waking hour.

Protein drink (recipe on Page 96):

- Drink one cup an hour after rising, then one cup every 2–3 hours as needed. If you like the taste of vegetable juice, use that for the basis of your drink instead of fruit.

Supplements

Probiotic	Morning and evening
Magnesium	150 mg morning, noon, and evening
Multivitamin-Multimineral	As directed on the label
Omega-3 Fatty Acids	3 grams of fish oil, flaxseed oil, or a combination
Fiber	Soluble fiber added to drinks 2 to 4 times per day; you don't have to add insoluble fiber to the protein shakes unless you want to because it changes the texture

The amount of fiber added depends on the type of protein drink and whether it has fiber added; the goal is 15 to 25 grams. If you'd rather not add fiber to your protein drink, simply use the regular fiber cocktail three times a day.

Before You Start to Detox

There are questions that always come up in any nutritional program. In this chapter, I'll answer the most common questions based on my experience. Please read this before proceeding with any phase of the program.

Should everyone try the cleanse or detox programs?
The answer is no. Some people with a chronic illness believe that by cleansing and detoxing their body, they'll get better control of their disease; that may or may not be true. The objective is to help you gain health benefits without putting yourself at greater risk. While there's no way to know precisely who should and should not do the program, here are some examples of those who shouldn't:

- Anyone who is underweight and malnourished. Your nutritional margin of error is much smaller because you have no reserves of nutrients. If your nutrition levels are adequate but you're naturally thin, that's acceptable.

- Women who are pregnant or nursing. This is not the right time for you to avoid food as you would with the cleansing fast—there's someone else depending on what you drink and eat for the nutrients needed to grow. When you're done nursing, that's a good time to do cleansing. I specifically used the word cleanse, not detox; with the detox program, you should get plenty of calories so it's not a concern. Because the foundation is eating only vegetables and fruits for two days out of 270 days, detoxing should be fine, but check with your doctor to be sure.

- Anyone undergoing treatment for a life-threatening disease. This is a time when you need all your energy to heal and get healthy. You shouldn't restrict calories because it can affect how well the treatment works. Even the Part Two section on fasting is experimental at this point, and we don't know how it might work with every life-threatening disease.

- Anyone who has recently had major surgery or is going to have major surgery. Again, you don't want to restrict calories because it can affect the efficacy of the treatment. You need to prepare for surgery by being as nutritionally stable as possible. Even though you have a short fast before surgery so food doesn't interfere with anesthesia, you don't want to be calorically depleted from reducing food intake for too long. Recover first, then try the program.

- Anyone going through a major life change. If you're moving to a new home, starting a new job, getting a divorce, grieving a loved one, or facing any highly stressful event, this isn't the time to experiment with a different way of eating. Focus on eating healthier, wait until your life has evened out a little, and then start.

There are other conditions that may warrant waiting to do the program, but the reasoning behind these recommendations is simple: one major stressor at a time is plenty for your body to deal with. While the outcome of the program should be a positive one, it's stressful to the body and should be done only with limited health challenges. As for the everyday stress of life, it isn't going away anytime soon so it shouldn't stop you from doing the program.

Should I check with my physician before doing the program?
Absolutely—if you have pre-existing conditions or are taking

medications, your physician may not agree with the concept of cleansing or detoxifying. That's fine. But if you want to do it, you need his or her assistance in adapting the program to your current drug regimen or physical state.

For example, your doctor can tell you whether it's safe for you to take your medications without eating if you want to do the cleanse. If you must consume calories while taking medication, do it. Whether you use the protein drinks or one of the detox soups, you can get calories safely while you take your medications and still accomplish your objective of improving the way your body functions.

Are there any foods or drinks I should avoid?
Yes: alcohol. We want to enhance the way the liver processes toxins, and alcohol is a toxin. But beyond that, you don't really have to avoid caffeine, artificial sweeteners, or food additives such as colors and preservatives. The reason that you don't have to go out of your way to limit those is because they aren't part of the foods and drinks you'll be eating during either the cleanse or the detox.

However, you can use The Elimination Diet for dealing with those types of substances. Fasting for two days really won't allow you to get a good handle on how problem foods might be affecting you. The Elimination Diet is designed to do that exact thing.

Should I be concerned if I'm spending extra time in the bathroom?
Not necessarily. You may have loose stools—some people associate that with diarrhea, but it's not the same thing. Your bowel movements may be different and more frequent than what's normal for you, so don't start the detox when you don't

have access to a bathroom, such as a camping trip. Save it for a weekend when you're at home.

Can I do the cleanse or the detox for only one day?
Yes—there's no single correct way to do this. I think two to three days is the right amount of time. But once you have experience with a single day and find out it isn't so bad, you can plan to do a two-day cleanse or detox next time. One day is better than none.

How often should I cleanse and detox?
How often you cleanse and detox depends on your nutritional lifestyle. The ultimate goal is to feel better and be healthier. If you consistently eat a healthy diet, you can do it less frequently—maybe four times per year. If you're in transition from a poor diet to a better one, cleansing and detox once a month may help you get your diet where you want it to be.

I understand what to do and why, but how am I going to feel during this process?
You won't know until you try—everyone responds in his or her own unique way. Here are phrases people have used to describe to me how they've felt when doing cleanses or detoxes:

Energized	Hungry
Light on my feet	Weak
Nauseated	Flatulent
Powerful	Enhanced sense of smell
Headachy	Clear thinking
Faint	Bad breath
Thinner	Sweet breath

You may feel some, all, or none of the above. The fact is that neither I nor anyone knows how you're going to feel during the process. But always keep this in mind: this is a voluntary process on your part. You can stop any time you want. There are no medals for gutting it out and no condemnation if you stop after half a day.

I'm diabetic—can I do the program?

Whether you're a type 1 or type 2 diabetic, you **must** discuss the program with your physician before beginning. Without a doubt, the foods are acceptable because they're healthy foods, but it's essential that you keep your physician informed of what you're doing and monitor your blood sugar regularly throughout the day.

What about my medications? Should I take them during the cleansing and detox?

Absolutely, and as stated earlier, you should check with your doctor about whether you must take them with food. You're trying to help your body work better with medications—that's one purpose of the detox. But **never** stop medications without talking to your physician.

Can kids do the cleanse or detox?

Children are not small adults—their metabolism is different because they're growing at a high rate. But once kids hit the teen years and are closer to adults in size, the program may be beneficial. If they're willing to eat the detox foods—cruciferous vegetables aren't big favorites with most kids—their bodies will benefit. I've included some modified recipes to make them more palatable to children when you move on to daily detox.

My doctor says that detoxification and cleanses are just a waste of time because the body does those things anyway. How do I respond?

The suggestion that occasional cleansing and detoxification aren't needed is based on incomplete data. Too often the assumption is that we eat the way people ate years ago when the only processed food was bread and it was often made at home. Today, it's unusual to eat foods that aren't processed and don't contain preservatives, added flavors, colors, and sweeteners. It doesn't mean they're bad, but in reality, we don't know how they affect our internal workings long term. Doesn't it seem logical to give our bodies a few days off from processing all those chemicals now and then? For more, read Chapter 7 in Part Two called "Are Cleansing and Detox Legit?"

The Detox Program

The goal of this detox program is to support the detoxification systems of the body by providing the right nutrients from food. How your body's detoxification system works is explained in Part Two. For now, here's what to do and how to do it.

There are several ways to take in the vegetables and fruit to support the detox process, but the most convenient way is in the form of soup. Fix a couple of the soups the day before, and you're set for a couple of days—or that's what I've thought until recently. What you lose is the sensation of chewing unless you make the soups chunky.

So I've added salads such as Broccoli-Cauliflower Salad and Coleslaw that add crunch and let you chew. Other ways of eating the vegetables and fruits are plain raw, slightly cooked, or even juiced.

While juicing has become very popular, I favor getting the entire plant material by eating the foods whole because the cellulose and fiber in the plant cells can feed the gut—but it's your choice. You can take the ingredients for any soup recipe and juice them, but I didn't test them that way so I can't guarantee the flavor. If you're an experienced juicer, you know what to add to improve the taste.

For this program, I'm sticking to soups and salads you can make in advance; then just heat them up or put them on a plate and you're done.

This detox program is very simple and lasts two days. Could you do it longer? Sure, but remember our premise. Real life. Two days off work. I definitely recommend starting on a

Chapter 4

weekend until you know how detoxing will affect your bathroom habits.

The Detox Program

This program is easy:

> **Eat as much as you want of any of the detox soups or salads or drink as much as you want of the detox drinks at any time on any schedule that fits your life.**

The same holds true for juicing, steaming, or lightly sautéing the vegetables. The only rule is that you should stick to the foods on the list with the exception of herbs. Aromatic herbs are the ones used for seasoning foods; they include the famous "parsley, sage, rosemary, and thyme" along with dill, basil, tarragon, and so on; chives can also count as an herb. There are no aromatic herbs that you need to avoid, so consider this a good time to experiment with adding herbs to vegetables and fruits to find which combinations suit your taste.

The basic ingredients in each of the detox soups and salads are cruciferous and allium vegetables. It doesn't matter whether you use just the basic Cabbage Soup or Coleslaw or mix the Squash Soup or Broccoli-Cauliflower Salad with it. Whenever you get hungry, eat some soup or salad.

In addition, because you may not want to start or finish your day with soup, you can have the phytonutrient-rich Berry Combo in the morning and evening.

Each recipe has been designed to provide plenty of the right vegetables to support the detox systems in your body. They're low in calories per serving but this program lasts two days, not indefinitely, and you have a specific purpose—to support your detox system. While you may ultimately want to lose weight, this isn't the way to do that. It's a good idea to start a weight loss program with a cleanse or detox to give yourself the sensation of feeling lighter and getting your head in the game, but then follow that with a reasonable weight loss program.

Recipes are in Part Three. A Detox Tracker to record what you eat is on Page 27, or you can download PDFs at www.drchet.com/real-life-detox. The last two columns are optional; see Page 44 for more info.

The Detox Drinks and Foods

The Detox Drinks

They're the same as for the cleanse: water, herbal tea, and green tea, as much as you wish throughout the day, hot or cold. The complete description is on Page 8.

Vegetables and Fruits

Use fresh or frozen; if you prefer organically grown vegetables and fruit, that's fine, too.

Cruciferous Vegetables:

Arugula	Kale
Bok choy	Kohlrabi
Broccoflower	Mustard greens
Broccoli	Napa or Chinese cabbage
Brussels sprouts	Radishes
Cabbage	Rutabaga
Cauliflower	Turnip greens
Collard greens	Turnips
Daikon	Wasabi
Horseradish	Watercress

Allium Vegetables:

Asparagus	Leeks
Chives	Onions
Garlic	Scallions
Green onions	Shallots

Fruits:

Black raspberries	Red grapes
Blueberries	Red raspberries
Dark cherries	Strawberries

The Supplements

Probiotic	Morning and evening
Multivitamin-Multimineral	As directed on the label
Omega-3 Fatty Acids	3 grams of fish oil, flaxseed oil, or a combination
Digestive Enzymes	15 minutes before eating, take the amount recommended on the label to help reduce any flatulence from the cruciferous vegetables

The Detox Tracker

Date _____

Time	What I Ate	Energy Level	Digestive Issues

Energy Level
1 – I need a nap.
2 – All I can do is sit, and it's tough to focus.
3 – I'm no ball of fire, but I'm able to function.
4 – I have the energy to do what I need to do at work and play.
5 – Top of the world! I feel like I can do anything—physical or mental.

Digestive Issues
1 – No noticeable issues
2 – Gas: belching
3 – Gas: flatulence
4 – Discomfort in my digestive system, but not painful
5 – Pain in the upper digestive system
6 – Pain in the lower digestive system
7 – Feeling constipated
8 – Diarrhea or loose stool

Real Life Continues: Daily Detox

Real-Life Detox is designed to get you headed in the right direction when it comes to the foods you eat. The Cleanse and Detox sections fit into real life—you know, the one that has kids, jobs, businesses, family, homeownership, and on and on? *That* real life. But what do you do now? Go back to your old way of eating, whatever that was? I would hope not.

What should you do next? You could try to become a vegetarian, eating only organically grown foods. Odds are it wouldn't work because it's an extreme lifestyle change that won't fit in your real life. But what you can do is take a few elements from what you've done during the detox program and put them into your everyday life. The idea is to build a new way of eating and drinking one building block at a time instead of a wholesale change. Let's take a look at some of the things that you could add to your life to gain benefits from what you've learned.

Drinks

Green Tea
Adding green tea to your diet every day can provide you with great phytonutrients and the potential for real health benefits, such as a reduced risk of some diseases such as cancer and heart disease, weight loss, and a reduction in cholesterol. Simply drinking green tea won't overcome a diet of highly refined foods, but it's one building block in the process.

Water
My personal belief is that people run around dehydrated more than they realize. Some of the benefits they feel in their digestive system during the Cleanse and Detox could simply

because they have more fluid in their systems. That means the blood runs thinner, carrying more oxygen to the body, and there's enough fluid in the digestive system to prevent constipation—two of the major issues that people say they face. Wouldn't it be ironic if it was simply a matter of drinking enough water that provided the most benefit?

Food

Cruciferous Foods
The detox recipes focus on cruciferous vegetables such as cabbage and broccoli. There's no reason that you couldn't focus on having one or two servings from one of the many recipes every day. I love coleslaw and can eat it every day. The same is true with the Broccoli-Cauliflower Salad. For you, maybe it's one of the soups or just plain raw veggies with a honey-mustard dip. If you eat those categories of foods every day, you will be detoxing every day without really doing anything special—it's just part of your eating plan.

Vegetables and Fruits
Make it a goal to get at least seven servings of vegetables and fruits every day—that's been shown to be the tipping point. If you can make that one change while including some of the detox foods, that will do more for your health than any other single thing you can do, with the exception of regular exercise.

I'm not going to tell you to stop all refined foods, fried foods, fast foods, regular soda, wheat, or any other foods or drinks. That's what everyone else tells you to do. Would that be a good idea? Probably—but I'm not going to eat that way, so how can I ask you to do something I'm not willing to do?

If you start your day with the goal of eating seven servings of vegetables and fruits per day, a few things will happen.

First, you're going to get the benefits from the vitamins, minerals, phytonutrients, fiber, and water in those foods.

Second, they're going to occupy space. As a result, you may not have the room to eat as much as you used to eat. Think about it. What if you ate an apple before you ate breakfast? What if you ate a salad loaded with lettuce, tomatoes, cucumber, and other veggies with just a plain vinaigrette before lunch? What if you had a serving of cabbage soup or coleslaw before you had dinner? What if you ate a banana before you ate a rich dessert? What might happen?

Third, you're going to change your diet to a healthier one, one that you can do in real life. That's the approach I've taken and continue to take. I could write another "eat a healthy diet and live forever" book, but the world doesn't need another one. All you need is to take what you've already learned and put it into your life one building block at a time. It won't turn your life upside down, and you can do it while you live your real life.

And there might be a fourth benefit: you may start to change the eating habits of your family and friends. Setting a good example of eating vegetables and fruit is great behavior to model for the kids in your life.

Take It Up One More Level

Based on the research I've done for this book, I'm going to be even more specific about the seven vegetables and fruits you should get every day. They may change over time as research reveals more, but for right now, this is how I would distribute the seven—have one serving of each:

1. Cruciferous vegetables of any type
2. Cabbage in any form, preferably raw as in coleslaw
3. Beans or legumes
4. Green leafy vegetables including every type of lettuce, spinach, watercress, and on and on
5. Any other vegetables; I prefer tomatoes—technically a fruit—because they're savory and have such great phytonutrients and flexibility
6. Berries of any type
7. Any other type of fruit

Here's a bonus: fermented foods provide additional bacteria that benefit your microbiome (more on that in Chapter 12). Fermented vegetables include fresh sauerkraut, kim chi, tempeh, and other vegetables. You're eating these to benefit your microbiome—your gut bacteria—so they can't be heated or the bacteria will be killed.

I know there will be questions such as "If I have two servings of sauerkraut, will that count as both the cabbage and the cruciferous?" Sure. Just don't overthink it too much.

Will this provide challenges to your digestive system and perhaps increase the gas you produce? Yes, but that should improve over time as your body adapts to the new diet, and you can always use a digestive enzyme. That's what I do.

Beyond that, there are no real rules to follow. Just give it a try and see what fits into your life. Every serving of vegetables and fruits you add is helping your body.

The Elimination Diet

Introduction

- Have you ever felt your energy drain after you're done eating a meal or snack?

- Have ever gotten constipated after eating?

- How about cramping and diarrhea?

- Do you walk around with a runny nose or watery eyes thinking, "I'm not allergic to anything—what's going on with these allergy symptoms?"

- Ever feel absolutely fantastic with energy to burn on one day, and the next day you don't want to get out of bed?

- Have you felt guilty because no matter what you do, you can't seem to will yourself to overcome it?

Did you ever stop to think that maybe those symptoms were related to what you've been eating—even if you don't have digestive problems?

That's what this chapter is designed to do: help you figure out whether these symptoms are related to specific foods you eat. We're going see if it's you or the food causing the issue, and the only way to do that is by using an elimination diet.

Is It You or the Food?

Should we care which one is the cause? Isn't the idea to just identify the foods so maybe we can feel better by simply eliminating them? I'm not trying to complicate something that seems simple at first glance: find the offender and eliminate it.

The problem is that it might be the food itself that's the offender or it may be the way your body is reacting to the food. Eliminating foods, either by entire groups or individual foods one at a time, is the only way of identifying *which* food causes the problem. *Why* it does is more complicated, and it's a question we may never get answered. That's okay because when we know which foods are the culprits, we can devise a strategy to deal with them so we feel better. Not all issues with foods are caused by the same process or system. Let's take a look at possible issues with the way our body handles foods.

Allergies, Intolerances, Genetics, and Unknown Factors

The classic symptoms of issues with foods relate to the digestive system: gas, bloating, diarrhea, constipation, and pain are among them. But the symptoms may have different reasons for different people. Let's take a look at each potential cause one at a time.

Allergies

If you're allergic to something, whether it's dust, pollen, or, in this case, some kind of food, it's going to trigger an immune response. Simply stated, it will cause an identifiable change in your immune system that results in the production of chemicals that say, "Hey—this is an immune response going on here!" If we were to obtain a blood test during that time, we would see that chemicals such as histamine and cytokines are increased. The culprit that started this whole problem is most likely immunoglobulin E or IgE for short. It became activated the first time you were exposed to that food. Nothing happened that time, but it primed your system for the next exposure.

Here are some of the symptoms associated with food allergies.

- Itching or swelling in your mouth
- Gastrointestinal symptoms, such as vomiting, diarrhea, or abdominal cramps and pain
- Hives or eczema
- Tightening of the throat and trouble breathing
- Drop in blood pressure

As you can see, your symptoms might be related to the digestive system with gas or diarrhea. But you may also get symptoms that are related to the typical immune response such as watery eyes and runny nose. The most serious example of an immune response is called anaphylactic shock: the throat closes and you have trouble breathing. If that ever happens, you need medical attention immediately!

The most common foods that cause anaphylactic shock are seafood in adults and nuts in children. The release of chemicals is so rapid and so extreme that the respiratory system can swell and prevent breathing.

Food allergies can occur anytime throughout your life, but children are the most susceptible. Why does this happen? No one really knows, but it most likely has something to do with the protein structures found in foods that set the IgE mechanism in motion. That's an oversimplification, but the result is that you have a food allergy.

The University of Nebraska, Lincoln Extension, suggests that peanuts, soybeans, fish, crustacea (shellfish), milk, eggs, tree nuts, and wheat are considered the most common allergenic foods on a worldwide basis. These eight food groups account for approximately 90% of all IgE-mediated food allergies and are sometimes referred to as the "Big Eight."

For now, the only solutions are to avoid these foods to eliminate symptoms or get allergy shots. If the symptoms are mild, you might be willing to endure them once in a while. But if they're severe, the foods should be avoided completely.

Intolerances
Food intolerances are caused by foods that for some reason we can't break down. The primary reason is generally the lack of the proper enzymes to break down the food, and the classic example is a dairy intolerance. Most people lose the ability to produce lactase, the enzyme that breaks down the milk sugar lactose. If you're one of those people who've lost that ability, you'll get gastric distress when you eat anything with milk sugar in it. This is different from a milk allergy. Let me explain.

With a dairy *intolerance*, you will be able to break down the proteins and fats in milk but you don't produce the enzyme to breakdown milk sugar; a dairy *allergy* means that you'll have a problem with any component of milk. That eliminates milk, cheese, and any product that's made with dairy. Again, it may be a matter of degree. You might be able to withstand cheese on pizza once in a while if the symptoms are minimal, but regular use could keep you in a bathroom for hours.

Another intolerance that's common is gluten intolerance, a protein found in wheat and some other grains. This is not the same as celiac disease, which I'll cover in Genetics.

One intolerance that we all seem to share is the intolerance to cellulose found in vegetables—this is especially true when it comes to beans. The most common symptom is gas. As the cellulose ferments in our digestive system, the bacteria breaking down the cellulose give off methane gas. You know the rest.

For now, there are no tests, genetic or otherwise, that can identify who is and who isn't prone to such intolerances; it's always trial and error, and that will be one of our objectives in The Elimination Diet. Any type of food is subject to temporary elimination if you think it may be a culprit. It may not result in gastric issues, but it may make you prone to fatigue and a lack of energy because it takes energy to deal with foods you're not digesting; in addition you may have poor absorption of other nutrients you need to make energy. Our goal is to have optimal energy to do what we want to do all day long and on into the evening; anything that may prevent the absorption of nutrients or takes more energy than it should to digest should be identified.

What's the solution? Once the food is identified, a broad-spectrum digestive enzyme taken before meals may allow a person to eat some of the foods; *broad spectrum* means it has enzymes to digest proteins, carbohydrates, and fats as well as cellulases to digest cellulose. Digestive enzymes may be effective in allowing a person to eat problem foods. If not—and not all digestive enzymes contain every possible enzyme—just as with allergies, the only solution is to avoid the foods completely.

Genetics
This is the most complicated part of issues with foods. There are estimates of 21,000 genes in our DNA. Some of them are activated together and can result in our inability to digest foods. The problem is that the only food-related genes we've identified are the ones that may result in celiac disease, the inability to digest gluten. With two genes, identified as DQ2

and DQ8, celiac can be predicted in parents and their children. However, there's still one more factor: whether those genes get expressed or not. Expressed means turned on; just because you have the genes doesn't mean they will be turned on. That's a serious complicating factor because you may live many years without any symptoms and then under the right environmental conditions, bam, the genes become activated. What activates the genes? No one really knows.

There are probably many more genes that are related to our inability to digest certain foods, but it will be years before they're all identified. Compounding the genetics is the whole idea of what turns the genes on. Seems like it's just easier to avoid foods that give you problems rather than worrying which category they fit into, doesn't it? Perhaps, but for me, I like to know the *why* even if the story isn't complete.

A new gene has been identified called transforming growth factor-beta, or TGF-beta. If this protein isn't expressed to a high level, it can result in several serious diseases such as Marfan's syndrome but can also contribute to severe allergies, including food allergies. There are years to go before we know anything substantive that can help us, but as I said earlier, it's complicated.

The only solution at this time is to avoid problem foods.

Unknown Factors
There are a couple of other factors to be considered when dealing with foods that don't fit into the other categories so I've called them unknown factors. There's no research on those substances to give us specifics on how they might contribute to our inability to digest foods.

The first and really obvious choice is probiotics, the good bacteria involved with the breakdown of foods. The problem is that there are estimates of as many as 5,400 varieties of probiotics living in our gut. We haven't identified them all and we don't know what they all do. That makes it difficult to recommend which one you or I might be lacking. It may be that bacterial balance may eventually lead the way to a permanent solution for our gut issues regardless of source. It's also likely it won't, but bacterial balance may help your body deal with some issues and foods.

Another unknown factor may be a metabolic disease such as type 2 diabetes. If you don't know that you have diabetes, you'll have a problem digesting carbohydrates, especially refined carbohydrates. While not a true digestive issue as others are, identifying how your body responds to carbohydrates of all types is important.

The Food

What we've considered up to now is our inability to digest foods for one reason or another, but the other part of that is the food itself. There may be characteristics within foods that cause us issues. If we don't know much about the genetics of food allergies, we *really* don't know much about the characteristics of the foods that can cause us problems. I'll give you some ideas but little is known. I should correct that. Little is known, but that doesn't prevent self-proclaimed experts from blaming the food.

The first culprit in today's world would probably be refined foods, which can mean anything from a loaf of bread to a cooked food such as soup in a can. You're not getting wheat, grinding it to make flour, and so on—you're buying a product that was prepared earlier. But the more highly processed the product, the more issues we can have with the food.

Whole wheat may be all right, but highly processed products may contain bleached flour—for instance some breads, cereals, and pasta that have virtually every nutrient removed and then put back in. On top of that, manufacturers are constantly looking for the ideal combination of fat, salt, and sugar to make us crave processed foods more. For more information, read *Salt, Sugar, Fat* by Michael Moss; while the tone of the book is written as an exposé of the food industry and how they strive to get us to eat more processed food, it's a fascinating revelation of how taste and flavor experts work behind the scenes.

Food additives would the next item on the list that may cause problems. That runs from substances such as monosodium glutamate (MSG) to artificial sweeteners to artificial flavors; manufacturers replace the natural flavors of foods with flavors made in a test tube. This is complicated because it may be a single molecule that's found inside the flavor or food enhancer, but it can still cause issues if you can't process it. This is not to say that these food additives are dangerous or unsafe. It simply means that your body can't process them for some reason, so you have to eliminate them from your diet.

But hold on. When you eliminate processed food and feel better, it might not be the component you think it is. You may think that it was the MSG or natural flavorings, whatever that really means, but it may be something else. The simplest action is to keep eliminating the food, especially if it's processed.

Another potential food issue is artificial colors. Many companies are turning to natural colors from foods because of the anti-artificial-color demands of consumers. While there have been issues in the past with colorings, colors available today have been tested and deemed safe. Again, that doesn't mean natural colorings won't bother you for one reason or another—you may have a problem with the source food—but it's something to consider.

Are you getting the idea that this is complicated? That's because it is. When your great-grandparents' garden offered just one type of potatoes, prepared one way in their own home, finding problem foods was easier. Today, just think about all the ways potatoes are processed and all the foods that contain potatoes—processed and with additives added to keep them shelf stable and safe so we don't get exposed to botulism or some other bad bacteria.

But the one that's probably on more people's radar is genetically modified organisms or GMO for short. Rather than use the process of normal plant husbandry and cross pollination, technology now allows scientists to take a gene with a specific trait such as resistance to certain bacteria and insert that gene into another plant; another example is a gene that confers the ability to make more of a nutrient, such as rice with more beta-carotene. But that's not all. Scientists have also inserted genes that will make wheat resistant to insecticides. And sometimes, they just want to make the food prettier so you'll buy more and less will end up in a landfill, which is also a worthy goal.

Is GMO bad? As of this writing, there's no research to suggest that it isn't safe, but this is a long road that's just begun. There's also no indication that you won't be allergic to or able to digest GMO foods. They could be a culprit for you.

Part of the problem with processed or GMO foods is the emotion associated with it. Whether it's the use of antibiotics in cattle, finely ground salt which hits your taste buds first and makes you crave more, or additives in foods, many people view this with emotion. Think about it like a business: no one is intentionally trying to develop products that kill or harm customers, because they want to keep every customer.

Food, whether organically grown or the most highly processed food you can imagine, is an issue that you can learn how to deal with in a very calm and cool way. It may be something as simple as a category of food that even grown organically, your body can't process—for example, nightshade plants such as tomatoes. That's just the hand you were dealt and no one is to blame. The Elimination Diet is the way to single out the foods that cause you problems. Now let's look at how you're going to get this done.

The Elimination Diet

There are many elimination diets out there in healthland. I'm certainly not going to suggest they're bad in any way because they do work, especially those designed to identify food allergies. The problem is that they're complicated in design. Basically, they have you eliminate potential problem foods all at once such as dairy, soy, or grains. With some plans, you have to stop eating everything except a bland food such as brown rice for a few days or a week to begin. Then, you start adding foods one category at a time.

I think it's too drastic to use that approach—and what if it's the brown rice that's causing your problems? It's just not practical in real life. Do you want to carry around a bucket of brown rice to eat at every meal? Do you want to completely throw out categories of foods that are not the culprit?

If we pay attention to how our body reacts to the foods we normally eat, we can be a little more concise in our approach to eliminating foods that bother us.

Let me give you an example from my life. I sometimes have a lag in energy either in the morning or the afternoon. Usually, a 20-minute nap and I'm good to go. But it doesn't happen every day. I don't like eating breakfast—I never have unless it's something such as biscuits and gravy on the weekend when there's nothing pressing to do. I eliminated breakfast, and my energy levels increased. If I'm hungry, I'll have berries and yogurt, which don't create an energy problem for me.

Thinking about lunch, I started to see a pattern. If I had bread or starches, such as a sandwich or something with pasta, I would need a nap. I could nap every day if I wanted to because I work at home most of the time, but it would be problematic under other circumstances. I also found out that when I'm driving long distances, I never get tired or sleepy if I eat only salads and fruit; but one burger and an hour later I can't keep my eyes open. I started keeping track and most of the time, the power drops were in relation to what I ate. I now save pasta and starches for the evening meals when I don't have much to do after eating.

By repeating the process with other foods, I found a cause for the watery eyes and sneezing that only occurred on some days. I love beer, especially one specific brand. If beer didn't have alcohol, I would drink it all day long. But I began to notice that I had itchy eyes and a runny nose in the morning after I drank beer. The problem would be worse if I had peanuts as well. This isn't the type of allergy or intolerance that's serious, but it can certainly be irritating. For me, the most important thing is to have optimal energy throughout the day. If it means peanuts, bread, and beer have to go, then unless it's vacation time—they go.

My point is that I didn't eliminate everything; I used a step-wise approach. I used trial and error with what I thought were potential suspects. I may have had a head start because of my expertise in nutrition, but I simply kept track of what I ate and how I felt during the following hours and days. In other words, I paid attention. I think with a little guidance, you can use the same approach.

Here's a three-step plan to identify problem foods. I like to use the example of a painter: begin with broad strokes, and when the foundation is laid down, then do the detail work.

Step One

For one week, write down what you ate from the beginning of the day until you go to sleep and the time you ate it; you don't need amounts at this point. There's a form you can photocopy on Page 47 and PDFs of that form and a larger size form are available at www.drchet.com/real-life-detox. Try to eat the foods that you normally would eat—this *isn't* the time to improve your diet. Jot down a note that you'll recognize such as "sandwich with turkey, lettuce, tomato, mustard." Write the time of day. Then track your energy level every hour along with any digestive issues you might feel. Whenever you eat anything, no matter how small, write it down: the time, food, energy level, and digestive issues that follow. It's important to continue to monitor energy and digestive issues because unless it's a severe allergy—which you may already know about—we're looking for changes that may be subtle.

For energy level, use a five-point scale found at the bottom of each page of the form:

> 1 – I need a nap.
>
> 2 – All I can do is sit, and it's tough to focus.
>
> 3 – I'm no ball of fire, but I'm able to function.
>
> 4 – I have the energy to do what I need to do at work and play.
>
> 5 – Top of the world! I feel like I can do anything— physical or mental.

For digestive issues, use this number scale for each symptom, and record each one:

1 – No noticeable issues

2 – Gas: belching

3 – Gas: flatulence

4 – Discomfort in my digestive system, but not painful

5 – Pain in the upper digestive system

6 – Pain in the lower digestive system

7 – Feeling constipated

8 – Diarrhea or loose stool

Step Two
Review the week. Look carefully at what you ate and the resultant changes in energy and gut issues. Then, after trying to see any patterns, pick one category of food from the list below and eliminate it for a week. Start with these largest categories of foods that seem to cause problems for many people:

1. Wheat such as bread and pasta

2. Corn and corn flour such as tortillas

3. Dairy such as milk, cheese, and yogurt

4. Eggs

5. Pork, beef, chicken, or fish

6. Anything else you noticed gave you an issue including carbonated beverages, tomatoes, whatever seems to cause problems; this is how I found out that pork gave me gas as flatulence.

The objective at this point is to eliminate that category of food for at least one week. Don't obsess about reading labels to see if there are any small amounts of each food; that's for later if you have to fine-tune things. For now, just pick one and eliminate it for a week while keeping track of what you ate. Record your energy level and digestive issues just as before.

Step Three
Add the eliminated food back into your diet while still keeping track. You're looking for patterns. If the symptoms had diminished or disappeared and then return, whether in energy levels or digestive issues, you have your culprit.

It may be a little more complicated than that. It may be the volume of the suspected food, the way it's prepared, or the way it's combined with other foods. If you don't care about the food, the simple approach is to eliminate it and you're done. But for example if you really love bread, you could try eating half the amount and see what happens. Or you could switch to whole grains or bread higher in protein or fiber. Or it may be that you simply can't handle the gluten protein in bread, and wheat flour is now something you can't eat without repercussions. Keep experimenting until you're sure.

At this point, you're done unless there's another food you notice is giving you an energy or gut issue. Then repeat the elimination process.

I think this approach to an elimination diet is better than throwing out large categories of foods—think of it as a selective elimination diet rather than a complete elimination-and-addition diet. By tracking how you respond to everything you would normally eat, you'll identify your suspects and how you respond by eliminating that single food.

The Elimination Diet Tracker

Date _____ Eliminated Food _____

Time	What I Ate	Energy Level	Digestive Issues

Energy Level

1 – I need a nap.
2 – All I can do is sit, and it's tough to focus.
3 – I'm no ball of fire, but I'm able to function.
4 – I have the energy to do what I need to do at work and play.
5 – Top of the world! I feel like I can do anything—physical or mental.

Digestive Issues

1 – No noticeable issues
2 – Gas: belching
3 – Gas: flatulence
4 – Discomfort in my digestive system, but not painful
5 – Pain in the upper digestive system
6 – Pain in the lower digestive system
7 – Feeling constipated
8 – Diarrhea or loose stool

Part Two:

Why You Should Detox

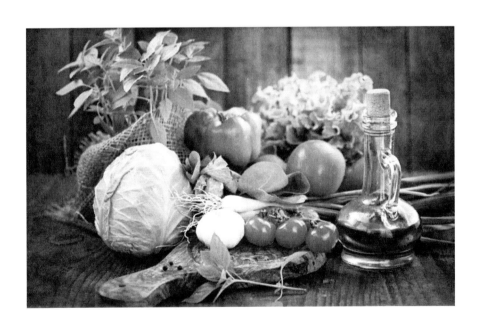

A Toxin Story

In the early 1970s, powerful toxins entered the food supply in the state of Michigan: a fire retardant called polybrominated biphenyl (PBB) was accidentally mixed with animal feed. Fire retardant is a good addition to many items, but it's not something you want in your food. This was a particularly nasty toxin for any living thing. How it happened is not exactly clear, but instead of supplementing cattle, chicken, and pig feed with magnesium, the feed was supplemented with PBBs. The results were catastrophic to the animals and subsequently the humans who ate the foods from those animals before the problem was discovered.

Because the animals' exposure was so vast, many of them developed significant health problems of the skin, kidneys, liver, and other organs. The source of the problem wasn't determined for a year; during that time, people in Michigan ate the eggs, milk, and meat from the animals. Were other areas of the country affected? The food tracking system wasn't as sophisticated then as it is now; there's no evidence the problem did spread to other areas, but no proof it didn't.

Just like the animals, people were exposed to the PBBs and had immediate health issues such as skin rashes, hair loss, and joint pain. Emory University has taken over tracking the people that were exposed to examine long-term health effects.

Once the cause of the contamination was discovered, the animals were destroyed. The economic cost to the state's farming economy was devastating. But that's not where our story ends—that's where our story begins.

You see, PBBs are fat soluble; that means they're stored in the fat cells of humans as well as animals. When we ate the animals, we ate the PBBs or the breakdown metabolites of PBB in the animals. Studies also indicate that the PBBs are excreted very slowly—researchers estimate that it would take 60 years to reach a level below one part per billion, the acceptable safe level. That implies there is a safe level, but that's never been established.

Sixty years! That means we're just now getting to the point where the PBBs are in the final process of elimination for those who were exposed.

The one thing that we know today is that we've been exposed to dozens if not hundreds of toxins from herbicides, pesticides, petroleum by-products from plastics, solvents, minerals such as lead, and many, many more in the air we breath, the homes we live in, the cars we drive, and the places we work. Something as innocuous as the markers we use on whiteboards or the off-gassing of the new carpeting we put in our homes are sources of chemicals that must be dealt with by our body's detoxification system on a regular basis.

While we have no significant examples of toxin exposure to humans through food since the event in Michigan, some of the toxins we're exposed to today are fat soluble and stay with us for long periods. We may be able to more quickly eliminate those that are water soluble, depending how effectively our detoxification system is working.

The obvious solution is to avoid all potential toxins—effective, but not realistic for those of us who live and work in modern society. If you can't avoid exposure, what do you do? That's what this book is all about: detoxifying your body in the real world we live in today.

Are Cleansing and Detox Legit?

I'm sure you've seen the ads for cleansing programs with people standing over toilets with long sticks holding up what they just eliminated. Gross, I know, but the reason it's offensive to me is that it's just not reality. The ads claim that this is what was caked in their digestive system, and this miracle cleansing program helped eliminate this sludge.

Bull.

These kinds of ads and claims give cleansing and detox a bad name. The main reason is that nothing builds up in your digestive system in the way they describe it—it's not physically possible. That doesn't mean that people don't overeat to the extent that their digestive system is never really empty, but nothing adheres to the walls of the digestive system. In addition, the cells of the small and large intestines turn over about every 72 hours. There's just no chance for a build up as described in those ads.

Why do people believe it? Because people *are* too full. People *do* feel bloated. It seems like a reasonable explanation. Well, it's not.

What is true is that we eat too much and never give our digestive system a break. In the U.S. and other modern countries, we're still eating mass quantities of high-fat, high-protein, and highly refined foods that challenge our digestive systems in ways other, simpler foods do not.

That's why clearing out our system once in a while is a good idea. Remember—we don't have the natural periods of feast and famine any more, so it rarely happens that our digestive tract is empty. I'm not talking about starving yourself; I'm just suggesting that giving the digestive system a break, like pushing the reset button, isn't a bad thing.

Cleansing

Let me give you an example. Ever have the flu? The kind where you have things coming out both ends, and the most you can choke down is water and a few saltines? Two or three days and you're back at it. The flu was horrible, you're hesitant to eat much, but a few days after all the trauma, your digestive system feels pretty good. You may have lost several pounds, but the farther you are from the symptoms of the flu, the better you feel—even though you haven't eaten for a few days. Was it pleasant? No, but you did what a cleanse is supposed to so: go through a period of eating no solid food. There's nothing magical about it. It's the way the body works.

Is there any evidence that cleansing programs work? No direct clinical trials have been done as of this writing.

Let's look at this two ways. First, can the colon be cleansed? If you've ever had a colonoscopy, you know the answer. Clear fluids for a day combined with a laxative such as magnesium citrate or polyethylene glycol will clean out your colon, without a doubt. Often, the last step is an enema. When they put that tube with the camera in your colon to look around, you're empty.

The second question: are you actually healthier after that? It depends on what your definition of healthier is. If you feel healthier when you feel lighter and have the empty feeling I described with the flu or food poisoning (minus the vomiting and diarrhea, of course), then the answer is *yes*. Has anything else happened that will enhance your health? Not really, but that depends on what you do next. You'll learn more about that in the following chapters.

Let me say a word about enemas and a more elaborate process called colonic irrigation or colonics for short. Colonics have used coffee as the fluid and in researching the topic, rectal burning because the coffee was too hot is frequently mentioned. Unless you really need an enema because of a health issue such as prolonged constipation, I'm not in favor of using them regularly. I also see no reason to get colonic irrigation for one simple reason: colonics have the potential to disturb the good bacteria called probiotics, often referred to as the intestinal flora. Your body contains 100 trillion or more, so you're not going to get rid of all of them, but you can upset the natural balance. But if you still believe that having someone shove a tube up your butt and rinse your colon with coffee is healthy, send this book back to me and I'll refund your money. It's just not necessary.

Detoxification

Detoxification programs are often promoted as cleansing the colon in combination with a myriad of foods, juices, herbs, or other concoctions that will remove toxins from the body, ranging from naturally occurring harmful chemicals to man-made substances. There are also other types of detoxification that involve sweating, foot baths, and foot pads.

These programs are what give detoxification a bad name. Detoxification is the real deal, and your liver can do it if you provide it with the right nutrients and support.

But the question is this: is there any research to support a detoxification program? There are no double-blind, placebo-controlled trials to be found by medical-research search engines. So how do we know that legitimate detox programs work? We don't—directly, that is. But there have been many clinical trials on animals that demonstrate that specific nutrients will cause the detoxification enzymes to work more effectively.

For the most part, traditional medicine doesn't recognize cleansing or detoxification as relevant to health. Maybe it's the way physicians are trained: something is broken, let's fix it! Don't get me wrong; if I need heart surgery, I want the most skilled surgeon in the world fixing it, and I don't care if she believes in cleansing or detoxing. Same is true for other types of surgeries, infections, cancer treatments, and on and on. That's what physicians are good at, and we should all be grateful for them.

But while they have been trained in how to deal with a thyroid that's underactive or a pancreas that no longer makes enough insulin, they get very little training in helping people obtain optimal health. The absence of disease doesn't mean someone feels great, has enough energy, and has all organs in their body working with peak performance. On several medical organization websites, the concept of detox programs is dismissed as unnecessary. Here's one such quote: "The idea that your body needs help getting rid of toxins has no basis in human biology." And "Your organs and immune system handle those duties, no matter what you eat." Remember those words: "no matter what you eat."

Supermarkets carry an average of more than 38,000 different items on their shelves. The Pew Charitable Trusts' Food Additives Project estimates that there are more than 10,000 chemicals allowed in food that help make this variety possible. These chemicals perform many functions, including enhancing the taste or appearance of food, preventing spoilage, and aiding in packaging the products. Here's the key point: in order to eliminate the chemicals that are a part of the modern diet, your body is going to use the same detoxification system that eliminates pharmaceuticals. Physicians certainly understand that's true because they guard against some combinations of medications or medication and food. Why? The detoxification required by either the medications or foods may conflict and cause serious problems.

To some degree, I think physicians read the same ads everyone else reads; they skim them and determine that they're absurd. I don't blame them for that, but I do blame them for not checking further. Most seem to view detox as an attempt to lose weight rapidly and most especially in an unsafe way by fasting for several days or by taking herbal concoctions that have never been studied in double-blind, placebo-controlled trials. Many seem to have a fixed mindset about traditional medicine being the one and only path to health.

Except nothing about traditional medicine is about obtaining optimal health. Have you ever had your doctor ask you to come to the office for a wellness examination where he will examine your diet to recommend improvements, walk you through a stretching and strengthening program, and teach you some tips and tricks for lowering your blood pressure or cholesterol?

Not in this lifetime—no health insurance company would pay for that. I know many physicians are frustrated by the stranglehold insurance companies have on how they can practice medicine, but they have no choice; they have to work within the system as it is now.

And yet, most people trust their physicians above just about everyone else. I can't tell you the number of times I've heard, "My physician told me..." and it's either that way or the highway.

It's the great irony of modern medicine: physicians have their patients' trust, but they don't have the time to use it. Yet they have no problem criticizing an approach to a healthier lifestyle that isn't mainstream.

Cleansing and detox are legit. It may be years before the randomized controlled trials are done, but based on the way individual components of the digesting system work, there's enough good science to support cleansing and detox as described in this book. Of course, none of that matters if cleansing and detox work for you—and you won't know that until you try them for yourself.

Fasting: Your Body's Reboot

When you use one of the cleansing programs using no- or low-calorie liquids, you're actually fasting. Some might argue that eating fewer calories than you need, such as when you follow a reduced-calorie diet, is also a fast, but that's not how we're defining a fast in *Real-Life Detox*: a fast is no solid food for specified periods of time. The length can vary, but 24 to 48 hours seems to be optimal based on research.

Some people restrict calories for religious reasons. For example, during Ramadan, people who follow Islam don't eat or drink from sunup through sunset. Mormons fast for two consecutive meals while focusing on their spiritual life. But that's not the idea in *Real-Life Detox*.

Fasting is an intentional withholding of calories to obtain potential health benefits.

Fasting stresses the body and it stresses the mind. When you're intentionally fasting for two full days, you know that you can eat at any time—you just choose not to. That's a psychological stressor. At the same time, you're stressing the body by not eating solid food while you maintain fluid levels.

Fasting isn't just a fad; it can have real health benefits. At the same time, it has become somewhat faddish. At least one book has been written that recommends alternate days of fasting and eating. Some diet plans manipulate the times for eating to try to obtain benefits by not eating for 12 to 18 hours. There may be merit to stopping the digestive process for those lengths of time, but it's probably not long enough to gain the complete benefit of fasting for one or two days.

The Premise

My premise for fasting is based on what our ancestors naturally endured. Food was not available on a regular basis even after we learned how to raise crops and animals. As a result, those who could live for days or longer without food survived and those who couldn't died. Our genetic code may be—and I say *may* be—hardwired for us to go through periods of feast and famine. The problem in modern society is that there has not been a famine in several generations. With food constantly available, famine doesn't exist unless we intentionally allow it, and I believe that has greatly contributed to the current obesity problem.

Don't misunderstand me—I'm not saying we should intentionally not grow food to feed ourselves and the rest of the world just to induce famine. There are still too many areas of the world that face famine every day and too many people here who go hungry. What I'm suggesting is that we may be able to gain some real health benefits by fasting for a day or two every few months and utilizing the famine-induced genes provided by our ancestors.

There's a lot of research on various types of fasting, but there's no consensus on what constitutes a fast; it ranges from missing one meal to indefinitely reducing caloric intake by one-third in an attempt to extend life. Therefore, the research isn't as precise on exactly how we can benefit from fasting.

Let me give you an overview of a recent research report that illustrates the potential benefits of fasting. The definition of fasting was no food for two to five days. The researchers believed that approach was more beneficial because it depletes muscle glycogen, the body's usual source of fuel. The body must then switch to other fuel sources: fat and ketones, breakdown products of fat. That length of fasting in mice and humans caused the immune system to essentially regenerate itself. In the process, it shifted stem cells from a dormant state to a state of self-renewal; the body got rid of non-essential substances, including worn out white blood cells. After the mice and people started eating again, the blood cells, and thus the immune system, were replaced with new and healthier cells.

It's a bit like rebooting your system. When your computer starts acting weird or the apps aren't working right on your phone, you know it's time to reboot—turn it off and then turn it back on. Usually your phone or computer work normally after a reboot. It's an over-simplification, but fasting seems to serve a similar purpose in our bodies, and every now and then, it's good to reboot.

There's a long way to go before the mechanisms of fasting are completely understood and the benefits established, but that doesn't mean we have to wait to try this process on ourselves. Remember that your body is unique, and what works for someone else may not work for you. A short fast may turn out to be great, in which case you've helped your body renew itself. It may turn out to be not as great and you've been hungry for a couple days and simply emptied your digestive system. You won't know until you try.

Use the approach in the cleansing programs and expect to see a healthier digestive system after the cleansing fast—no miracles promised. But if the market works as it usually does, I predict there will be fasting programs developed implying there are amazing benefits to your body, renewed immune systems, cures for all kinds of diseases, and on and on. Building a program that makes outlandish claims based on a study or two is lame, but it happens all the time. Just remember when you see an ad for a miracle fast online, you already know what the research says and you've got all the info you need right here.

I believe fasting is beneficial for our bodies, and it's worth the effort to fast for two days every couple of months. The truth is that no one can guarantee that the benefits will occur for everyone, or for anyone for that matter. Current research indicates that short fasts are good for your health; if that changes, I'll be sure to let you know.

The Science of Detoxification

Detoxification is the process of eliminating natural and man-made toxins from the body; it's something our body does naturally if we eat a diet full of the right nutrients. Those nutrients include vitamins, minerals, and phytonutrients; other nutrients such as omega-3 fatty acids and amino acids may contribute to the process and support the vegetables and fruits.

And that seems to be the issue in modern society: our poor diet, with so many refined foods, contains a multitude of chemicals, which may be overwhelming our detoxification systems. While detoxification is completely natural, it doesn't work well in most people. So for our purpose, we'll define detoxification as refreshing and restoring the biochemical systems in the body. The idea is that removing toxic substances from our bodies can help us feel better and improve our health. To that end, let's look at the science of detoxification.

The liver is the most important organ in the detoxification process. Other organs are involved—the digestive system absorbs nutrients and then eliminates some toxins, and the kidneys eliminate other toxins—but the bulk of the work is done in the liver.

Potential Toxins

Obviously, avoiding exposure is the best scenario, but that's not always possible depending on where we work and play. Here are the categories and some of the substances that are in those categories:

Metals
These include arsenic, cadmium, lead, mercury, nickel, tin, and so on.

Inorganic Substances
Asbestos, carbon monoxide, and hydrogen sulphide are in this category. Carbon monoxide is made up of one carbon molecule and one oxygen molecule, while asbestos is a complex natural chemical compound containing atoms such as potassium, sodium, magnesium, aluminum, silicon and others; each atom individually might not be harmful, such as carbon or magnesium, but when combined into complex compounds can be toxic.

Hydrocarbons
Both natural and man-made chemicals, including propane, butane, pentane, and hexane.

Aliphatic Alcohols, Ketones, Ethers, Aldehydes, and Acids
Some examples you might recognize are ethyl alcohol (ethanol) found in alcoholic beverages and acetone found in nail polish remover.

There are many more categories that would fit into the man-made chemical category such as pesticides and dioxins used as coolants in electrical transformers.

One of the factors that makes these substances more problematic is that many are relatively new. Think back to pre-historic times; humans burned wood for heat and cooking, warning away predators, and so on. Theoretically our bodies had many, many generations to learn how to counteract the toxins from wood smoke. But many man-made chemicals have been around only one or two generations; our bodies haven't had much time to develop coping mechanisms. Choosing to detox may be even more essential now than in the past.

The point is this: there are many harmful toxins that we are exposed to on a regular basis. If the body can eliminate them, it's by using the detoxification system in the body.

The Detoxification System

The liver is the most important organ in the natural detoxification process of the body and does the job with enzymes, proteins that speed up chemical reactions. There are two enzyme systems in the liver to detoxify the body: the phase 1 and phase 2 detoxification systems.

Phase 1 Detoxification
The phase 1 detoxification system is responsible for eliminating fat-soluble substances from the body, substances that are not soluble in water but only in fat. That means they can't be eliminated via the digestive system because they're in the liver, and they can't be eliminated via the kidneys unless they're transformed into water-soluble substances. The chemicals that are fat soluble and must be transformed include medications, pesticides, food additives, alcohol, and other contaminants. The phase 1 enzymes transform most of these substances from fat soluble to water soluble.

Phase 2 Detoxification
Along with other water-soluble toxins, phase 2 eliminates the now-processed chemicals from phase 1. Fat-soluble substances have been converted to water-soluble substances and can be eliminated through urine, sweat, and feces.

Both detoxification systems can be enhanced by eating the right foods and eliminating some stimulants and food additives. The only elements I've found in the research that consistently help our body detoxify itself are two categories of plant foods: the sulforaphane class and the allium class.

Sulforaphane foods include those such as cabbage, broccoli, cauliflower, bok choy, and many other cruciferous vegetables. While sulforaphane works in both phase 1 and phase 2, it's used more in the phase 1 system.

The allium-containing foods are in the onion-and-garlic class of foods and are primarily used in the phase 2 system. Add foods such as antioxidant-containing fruits with vitamin C, and you have the foods that help your liver detoxify your body. If you eat them every day, your liver and entire body get the benefit.

The Complexity of a System

I would not be doing you a service if I led you to think the detoxification process is as simple as I just explained. That's probably a deep enough understanding for the layperson—I don't want your eyes glazing over—but keep in mind that it's much more complicated. Let me give you a couple of examples.

We know that your genes play a significant role in how the detoxification process works in your body. For the most part, there are no commonly available genetic tests to tell whether you have any of the many single-nucleotide polymorphisms (SNP) with variants of the same gene. We don't know whether one SNP ("snip") could interfere with the detox process or whether it would require many SNPs. We also don't know exactly what would express these genes (turn them on) or what would down regulate them (turn them off) and whether the order those were done would make a difference. Getting the idea that this is complicated?

Let me give you an example of how complex it might be. One of the toxins many of us intentionally expose ourselves to is alcohol. We might think that it would be a good idea to eat more cruciferous vegetables while we drink, with the idea that it would help detox our liver even as we were imbibing. Maybe, maybe not.

In a study done in Finland, researchers isolated one of the phytonutrients from cruciferous vegetables called phenethyl isothiocyanate (PI). They administered it to rats along with alcohol for several weeks. For the most part, the PI produced the expected benefits of protecting the liver, but a breakdown product of alcohol metabolism called acetaldehyde was raised to high levels. If susceptible individuals, whom we cannot yet identify by their genes, were to eat high levels of cabbage or other cruciferous vegetables while they were drinking, they could get deathly ill. I don't mean they would die, although it's possible—I mean they would want to die because of the severe vomiting and headaches brought on by the combination of cruciferous and alcohol. For that select few, the traditional green beer, corned beef, and cabbage on St. Patrick's Day are probably not a good idea.

Understand, this is possible but we don't know how likely. Remember, researchers used a concentrated amount of one phytochemical from the cruciferous vegetable; with the actual vegetable and all its other nutrients, it might not happen at all. But this illustrates how complex the detoxification system is.

It also illustrates another important point: look for your nutrients from foods first, then whole-plant concentrates before you look at concentrated nutrients of any type. There's a reason that vegetables and fruits developed their particular distribution of beneficial nutrients, and our bodies have adapted to that complex mix. When we take a single extract as the solution to our problems—even with the best intentions—it may have unintended consequences. Food first, people.

It's the Bacteria, Stupid!—A Theory

If you're old enough to remember Bill Clinton's first presidential run, you may remember campaign director James Carville's blunt response to a campaigner's question on what the campaign was about: "The economy, stupid!" After thinking about the role that the foods I've covered mean to the detoxification process, something seemed so obvious that I wrote down: The bacteria, stupid! I'm referring to what we used to call the intestinal flora but today is more commonly called the microbiome. Based on the available research as of this writing, as goes your microbiome, so goes your health.

Micro what? Microbiome. This is the most recent term to describe the 100 trillion or more microbes that live in and on our bodies; microbes are organisms too small to be seen with the naked eye. A single clear definition hasn't been agreed upon, but according to the American Academy of Microbiology, "The human body hosts a huge number of microbes of many different kinds. These microbes play a role in many fundamental life processes. The collection of microbes that constitute the microbiome is not random; the human microbiome is made up of a particular set of microbes that complement each other and the human host." The whole report is fascinating, and I recommend it to anyone who wants to more fully understand the microbiome; info on how you can find the report is in the References.

By calling this collection of bacteria and other microorganisms the intestinal flora, we seem to be implying they're plants and they're most definitely not; it also suggests they're in the intestines, when they're actually everywhere throughout our bodies. The human microbiome includes several types of microorganisms, but for simplicity's sake, we'll stick to calling them bacteria.

So our working definition of the microbiome is this one: a collection of bacteria that inhabit the human body.

Diet Composition and the Microbiome
Why would I say that it's the bacteria? There are many factions within the nutrition community who believe they have the solution to a healthy 21st-century diet. From the traditional low-fat approach to the very-low-carbohydrate approach advocated by the current Paleolithic Diet faction, everyone finds research to support their position. Another faction is the one opposed to refined and processed food; they blame the food industry for making foods that hook us on sugar, fat, and salt. Even the vegans who avoid all animal products jump into the fray and try to show that all animal protein is bad for health and environmental reasons.

They're all right and they're all wrong—there are elements to each that may be correct. But the reasons may be wrong. Let me explain.

The low-fat advocates have demonstrated that they can reverse severe blockages in arteries; the programs of Dr. Dean Ornish and Dr. Caldwell Esselstyn have shown amazing results. The problem is that whether it's today or 200 years ago, it's a difficult way to eat. The lack of healthy fat from short- to medium-chain triglycerides as well as protein is difficult to sustain. Proteins are integral to the immune system staying strong as we age, and a low-fat diet may reduce the amount of protein available just at a time the immune system starts to deteriorate. Still, as I'll talk about later, the dependence on vegetables and fruits is beneficial to the microbiome.

The low-carbohydrate factions fall into two categories: those who want to eliminate refined food and those that want to reduce carbohydrates while increasing protein and fats. In the case of the anti-refined foods group, they look at the calories, sugar, and salt as the problem. In reality, it may be the additives in food that prevent the microbiome from functioning properly.

Let me explain it this way. Very few foods, whether animal or plant sourced, are what our ancestors ate 100 years ago: we grow our food for flavor, not nutrition. Changing the nutrition levels of beef by feeding the cattle corn instead of grass changes not only the fat content but also the types of fat. Growing corn that's super sweet changes the phytonutrient content. Look at any plant source of food, and it has been modified—and I'm not talking about genetically modified organisms. As soon as humans discovered crossbreeding, enterprising farmers started experimenting to discover better strains of plants and animals; that's just what we do.

However, the microbiome that could break down and process the nutrients 100 years ago may not have mutated to break down and process today's foods, even organically grown foods. Add the challenge from modern additives in refined foods, and the microbiome may not be able to function properly. Even though the detoxification process can eliminate the additives, it may stifle the growth of the microbiome, leading to an overall negative effect. On top of that, processing destroys all the bacteria on foods, even those that may be beneficial.

As for the Paleolithic Diet devotees, they just have it wrong. The diet was certainly modified over the many years until we began growing crops, but the foundation was always plant material. Paleolithic humans had to consume a lot of plants to get the protein they needed, because the available plants did not have a high protein content. Remember we're not talking about the wide variety of plants we have today—one culture lived primarily on a form of cactus. The fiber content of their diet was 150 to 200 grams per day! The typical person on a modern diet is lucky to get 10 or 15 grams. They certainly ate meat but were not the greatest hunters; meat was not a regular part of the diet until much later in that period, and that's a good thing. A high-protein intake stresses the microbiome and interferes with the normal growth of the good bacteria.

The reasons that every faction gives as the reason they have the healthiest diet might not be correct. It just might be that the healthiest diet is the one that focuses on feeding the microbiome the best. Now you're wondering if you could eat only fast-food burgers as long as you ate enough foods that provided healthy bacteria to the microbiome. That's a problem I'll cover in the next section.

Food and the Microbiome

Other than dairy foods with added cultures and fermented foods, there are no reliable lists of food sources containing the thousands of bacteria and other organisms that are found in our microbiome. Other than a fecal transplant from someone who has a healthy microbiome, there's no way to know where to get the many bacteria our gut needs. (Don't let the concept of a fecal transplant freak you out; it's much cleaner and less direct than you imagine. It goes like this. The feces collected from healthy subjects, or rather, subjects with a healthy microbiome, is cleaned and purified without killing the microbiome and is then transplanted into patients. It's becoming more common to treat inflammatory bowel disease but as of this writing, it's still an experimental procedure.)

Where you'll probably find good bacteria in the food supply is in raw fruits and vegetables. Organically grown produce is probably best, but there's no evidence that has proven it is; it simply makes sense based on the avoidance of chemicals during the growth process. It may be wise to shop the farmers markets for produce when available and shop in the organic section of the supermarket at least some of the time, but you're better off eating more of whatever produce you can find. Even the Environmental Working Group, a watchdog group that ranks vegetables and fruits according to the amounts of herbicides and pesticides, says it's more important to eat conventionally grown vegetables and fruit than to hold out for organic because the nutrients are more important than the chemicals they may contain.

What if it was never about the lack of chemicals or better nutrients in the organically grown vegetables? What if it was always the bacteria that made you feel better after eating organically grown produce? Wouldn't that be a hoot?

Where you will not find the bacteria you need is in the processed food that dominates our food supply. If the product was cooked or heated, the good bacteria were killed. Think of all the everyday foods that eliminates!

Your Microbiome Back-Up Plan

If you can't obtain effective amounts of good bacteria because your choices are so limited, you still have a good option: you can feed the bacteria you already have to help them grow and thrive. The way you do that is by eating more vegetables and fruit every day. Whether organically grown or not, they have fiber which nourishes the bacteria. This is especially true of inulin, a soluble fiber; it acts as fiber in the small intestine and then becomes a food source for probiotics in the large intestine. You could also limit your consumption of foods with added sugars such as those found in many refined carbohydrates. Research shows that they tend to feed the negative bacteria while leaving the good bacteria starving.

How many servings of vegetables and fruits are we talking about? The tipping point has been shown to be seven and if you can do ten a day, so much the better. Start with that amount of vegetables and fruits in your diet every day, add fresh herbs to pick up the additional good bacteria they can provide, and whatever else you eat may not matter that much.

DNA, Detox, and Your Genes

We're in the infancy of nutrigenomics, a field of science that examines how your genes interact with the foods you eat. It works both ways: your genes influence the way what you eat affects your body, and what you eat affects the way your genes behave. Feed your genes the right foods, and you're going to be healthier; feed them the wrong foods, and it may negatively impact your health.

But that's not all. There's another field called pharmacogenomics and as you might surmise, it's the study of how pharmaceuticals interact with genes. Your genes can affect how medications are processed—they can slow down the metabolism, speed up the metabolism, or have no effect.

But even that isn't all. Almost every gene has the potential to mutate over the years. Some mutations have no specific effect, while others can radically change the way foods and drugs are processed. The net effect is that the foods you've always eaten may affect you in a different way or the drug may not work as designed.

Aw, shucks, let's complicate things even further. The type of foods you eat and when you eat them can impact specific genes that process medications and also change their effectiveness.

To illustrate, let's look at one set of genes and their effects.

Cytochrome P450

These genes—the CYP 450s—are part of the phase 1 detoxification process, and they impact the phase 2 process as well. While they work primarily in the liver, they also work in other organs such as the intestines. They form a system of enzymes that catalyze chemical reactions to process many substances such as medications, foods, caffeine, and alcohol. It makes those substances water soluble so they can be eliminated. Pretty simple, right? Maybe not.

As of this publication date, there are about 60 known active CYP 450 genes in the human genome that have been sequenced, meaning scientists know their location and structure on human DNA. Each one of these CYP 450 genes has a slightly different role in the detoxification process. Scientists use short-hand to differentiate between the different forms of CYP 450 genes using letters and numbers such as CYP 450 1A2 and CYP 450 3A4.

Now it gets even better. There are mutations of these CYP 450 genes which change how they metabolize substances. The mutations are referred to as polymorphisms. If they affect just a single location on human DNA, they're called a single nucleotide polymorphism—a SNP. CYP 450 polymorphisms that have been identified may produce enzyme products with abolished, reduced, altered, or increased enzyme activity. Researchers categorize people with these polymorphisms into four groups (technically called phenotypes):

- Poor metabolizers: People with this polymorphism lack the functional gene altogether
- Intermediate metabolizers: They have one active form of the gene
- Efficient metabolizers: They have two active copies of the gene
- Ultrarapid metabolizers: They have more than two active forms of the gene

The net effect is that some medications may not work for some people at all because they don't have the gene to process it, or they process it too rapidly and it's eliminated before it can be effective.

How does this affect detoxification? CYP 450s also process substances in the foods we eat such as phytonutrients, caffeine, and alcohol. They can either help or hinder the detoxification process. Let's look at three different practical examples so you get a clearer picture of what this can mean.

Grapefruit Juice
If you take a medication such as a statin to lower cholesterol or verapamil to control irregular heartbeats, grapefruit juice can interact with the CYP 450 3A4 gene and affect the rate at which the medication is absorbed in the intestines. With statins, it may contribute to the muscle damage that can sometimes occur when people take that medication. But the important thing is only some people will have a problem—and we don't know who will and who won't.

Caffeine
This is important because some people (your author, for example) are dependent on coffee. Caffeine is metabolized in the liver by the CYP 450 1A2 into three different forms, each having its own effect on the body such as increasing fatty acids in the blood or dilating blood vessels. Research has shown that there are polymorphisms of this gene which can make some people fast metabolizers or slow metabolizers of caffeine. In one study, slow metabolizers who used caffeine regularly had an increased risk of heart attack compared with fast metabolizers.

What does this have to do with detoxification? It may be that for fast metabolizers, caffeine intake is of no consequence to detoxification and they can continue to drink it. It may also mean that slow metabolizers should avoid caffeine because it will take too long for their bodies to process it.

One more complication: the phytonutrients in green tea blunt the effect of caffeine in the body. So while coffee may have a profound effect on you, green tea—even with caffeine—may not because of a combination of all these factors.

Broccoli

The different phytonutrients in broccoli have been examined for their effect on some of the CYP 450 genes. In several studies, broccoli extracts have been demonstrated to kick-start both the phase 1 and phase 2 enzyme systems, thereby contributing to a chemoprotective effect. Bottom line: cruciferous vegetables contribute to the detoxification process and should be a part of all detox programs.

The Future of Detox

This is the state of the science as of this writing. Tomorrow, there will be more research to identify more genes and more interactions, both positive and negative, with the detoxification process. This program was designed using what we know today.

Most of the genes mentioned are not yet identified in the general public. In the future, you'll be able to base your total diet on information from your genetic code and detoxify yourself on a daily basis. Your diet will be specific to you.

Until then, I'm sorry, but you'll have to eat the broccoli!

What About Herbs?

If you've looked at cleansing and detox programs online, they always seem to have a variety of products that cleanse and detoxify including many herbal products. You might be wondering where they are in *Real-Life Detox*. I did extensive research on many herbs that are found in many of the cleansing and detoxification products; the list is at the end of this chapter, and it's extensive.

In reviewing the research, here's what I found. First, psyllium husks, flax seed, grapefruit pectin, and guar gum are fiber obtained from plants. Fiber is an important component of the cleansing program in *Real-Life Detox*. In my opinion, those are the critical ingredients of the cleansing products; the problem is that there isn't enough fiber in the available products to be beneficial.

The only herbs that seem to be beneficial for cleansing are those that act as laxatives: senna and aloe vera. The research shows that both are beneficial as laxatives and may help with constipation, but they're not critical to any cleansing or detox program. The goal is to restore natural digestive functioning, and unless these are herbs that a person is going to use every day, they aren't necessary in a cleanse. Medical oversight may be required if you have chronic constipation.

What about the rest of herbs on the cleansing list? There's no research to suggest that they're beneficial for cleansing. It doesn't mean that may not be beneficial for other reasons when used in the right quantities for specific conditions. But one of the characteristics of cleansing and detox products is that formulators seem to throw everyone into the pool, so to speak—maybe they're using every herb they can think of in hopes something will work, or maybe they're just trying to impress clients with the complexity of their product. However that's not the way we should approach cleansing our digestive system or detoxing our bodies—let's use what we know works and avoid the guessing game.

Are Herbs Essential?

You should understand that you never need to take an herb in your life. They're not nutrients that your body needs; they're not vitamins, not minerals, not good bacteria. They're not necessary for your body to function. If we're going to use herbs for cleansing or detoxing, we should use these criteria:

1. The herbal supplement must be backed by at least some research that shows benefits. It doesn't have to be perfect research or the most extensive, but there must be clinical trials on humans with a good result.

2. The herbal supplements must be standardized to the percentage of active ingredient shown to be beneficial based on research. That means you should buy from a company that has a scientific staff who knows the science, conducts research, and can assess the herbs to guide the manufacturer to make a product that will be effective based on the science.

3. Finally, buy your herbal supplements from a company using Good Manufacturing Practices to insure the products will not be contaminated, including monitoring where the plants are grown. There have been many issues with heavy metals in herbs from around the world, so regular testing for purity is important. We don't want to create more problems.

Herbs and Detox

The list of herbs used in detox formulations is as extensive as those in cleansing products. Again, sticking to the goal of restoring the detoxification system in the body, only two herbs have sufficient research to show they can be effective for that purpose. Garlic is an allium vegetable and as such, is important to the detoxification process. But in this case, I think using garlic in foods and cooking are a better way to get the phytonutrients from the garlic in a detox program.

The only herb that has satisfactory research in my opinion is milk thistle; it has been used to remove heavy metals from the body when given in standardized extracts intravenously. While beneficial, it doesn't need to be part of a detox program. It can be beneficial for specific conditions, but the purpose of this program is to get the natural detoxification system working well. What you eat and drink contributes more to that process than even a beneficial herb such as milk thistle.

What about the rest of the herbs on the list? While there have been traditional uses for most of those herbs, the effectiveness for each herb has not been demonstrated in human trials; thus the safety hasn't been established and potential for negative outcomes hasn't been eliminated. You might say, "But these have been used for 100s of years!" I understand that, but herbs in pills are not the same as the herbs that have been traditionally used. Your village healer didn't gather naturally growing plants from the woods and fields where you live; more likely they've been grown in a country with lax safety standards for the cultivation of herbs and other plants.

Herbs are closer to medicines than they are to foods. If you work with a naturopath who has training in the used of herbs and herbal blends, that's perfectly acceptable. But again, this approach of throwing everyone in the pool in the hopes no one will drown isn't a good idea in my opinion. Think about it. If we are concerned with vitamins or minerals and how they may affect medications, think about the potential interactions of 10 herbals in a single product when no tests for interactions have been conducted. Leave the herbs to the professionals. *Real-Life Detox* was designed to use real foods in your everyday life.

Just for fun, here's a list of most of the herbs I researched:

Cleansing Herbs

Senna leaf
Buckthorn bark
Fennel seed
Chamomile flower
Peppermint leaf
Cinnamon bark
Ginger root
Milk thistle seed
Rose hip fruit
Uva ursi leaf
Passion fruit

Psyllium husk
Flax seed
Papaya fruit
Grapefruit pectin
Slippery elm bark
Rhubarb bark
Guar gum
Alfalfa leaf
Licorice root
Aloe vera gel

Detoxification Herbs

Milk thistle seed
Burdock extract
Dandelion leaf and root
Fenugreek extract
Garlic extract
Lullein extract
Oat extract
Oregano extract
Stinging nettles extract

Turmeric extract
Bamboo extract
Natural chlorophyll
Cape aloe leaf powder
Rhubarb root
Marshmallow root
Slippery elm bark
Triphala blend

References

This reference list represents the important resources I used as a basis for writing *Real-Life Detox*. The list does not contain everything I read such as the references and citations in a research paper do. I did not include research I didn't write about. For example, I reviewed the research on over 40 herbs; that involved reading at least the abstract on dozens of published papers. The limited published research as well as the less than overwhelming results in clinical trials led me to conclude they were not necessary for this program.

This is a practical book that's to be used in your everyday life. It was never meant to be reference manual or a scientific text. This reference section reflects that.

Introduction

Cathy Copyright Universal Press Syndicate

Detox Program

7-Day Detox Miracle, Revised 2nd Edition: Revitalize Your Mind and Body with This Safe and Effective Life-Enhancing Program. 2001. Peter Bennett N.D., Stephen Barrie N.D. and Sara Faye.
This is the program for those who want to commit to detoxification for an extended period of time. It focuses on all aspects of detoxification, not just the physical. I would recommend it if you want to spend the time centering mind, body, and spirit.

The Elimination Diet

http://farrp.unl.edu/informallbig8

A Toxin Story

http://www.pbbregistry.emory.edu

Toxicological Profile For Polybrominated Biphenyls And Polybrominated Diphenyl Ethers. U.S. Department Of Health And Human Services Public Health Service Agency for Toxic Substances and Disease Registry. 2004.
This is the entire 600+ research papers.

Fasting

Prolonged Fasting Reduces IGF-1/PKA to Promote Hematopoietic-Stem-Cell-Based Regeneration and Reverse Immunosuppression Cell Stem Cell
http://dx.doi.org/10.1016/j.stem.2014.04.014
This is the article on fasting and the immune system; not easy to read, but it's an important research paper.

The Microbiome

http://academy.asm.org/index.php/faq-series/5122-humanmicrobiome
This is written by microbiome researchers for the general public to explain the human biome in detail; it's a must read for everyone who is interested in understanding the role of bacteria as well as fungi and viruses in health.

Some of My Best Friends Are Bacteria. Michael Pollan. NY Times 5-5-13.
This is written by a lay person and follows the writer's quest to better understand his gut bacteria.

Host lifestyle affects human microbiota on daily timescales. Genome Biology 2014, 15:R89 (25 July 2014)

Diet rapidly and reproducibly alters the human gut microbiome. Nature. 2014 Jan 23;505(7484):559-63. doi: 10.1038/nature12820.

Biosynthesis of vitamins and enzymes in fermented foods by lactic acid bacteria and related genera: A promising approach. Croatian J Food Sci Tech. 2013; 5(2):85-91.

J Pharmacol Exp Ther. 1995 Oct;275(1):79-83.
This is the study from Finland on cruciferous vegetables and alcohol.

Nutrition and Genetics

http://ghr.nlm.nih.gov/geneFamily/cyp.
The CYP gene family: a basic explanation of this family of genes

It's Not Just Your Genes! Ruth DeBusk and Yael Joffe. 2006. ISBN-10: 0977636305.
This is still the best book to explain how nutrition affects your genes; simple and easy to read with practical applications for your life. Regardless of your genetics, what you eat can make a difference to your health.

Part Three:

Detox Recipes

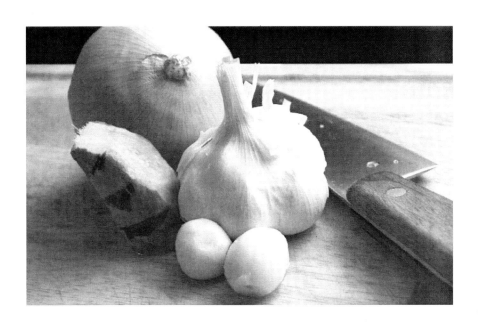

Recipes

The goal of the detox program and daily detox is to provide the nutrients that will enhance the phase 1 and 2 enzyme systems in the liver. That means plenty of cruciferous and allium vegetables:

Cruciferous Vegetables:

Arugula
Bok choy
Broccoflower
Broccoli
Brussels sprouts
Cabbage
Cauliflower
Collard greens
Daikon
Horseradish
Kale
Kohlrabi
Mustard greens
Napa or Chinese cabbage
Radishes
Rutabaga
Turnip greens
Turnips
Wasabi
Watercress

Allium Vegetables:

Asparagus
Chives
Garlic
Green onions
Leeks
Onions
Scallions
Shallots

Fruits:

Black raspberries
Blueberries
Dark cherries
Red grapes
Red raspberries
Strawberries

As stated earlier, you can eat these raw, juiced (all the edible parts run through a juicer), steamed, or lightly sautéed in olive oil or high-oleic safflower oil. One of the advantages of cooking these vegetables is that it reduces the strong flavor of the allium vegetables and some of the cruciferous. The choice is yours, but during detox make sure that you limit your intake to the vegetables on this list if you don't make soup.

Adapting the Recipes

As you will see, some of the recipes are modified and include a few things you wouldn't expect in a detoxification recipe: mayonnaise, sunflower seeds, oils, and so on.

During detox, stick to the basic recipes. But when you start to move these foods, especially the cruciferous vegetables, to your everyday life, you might want to modify them so they're more appealing, not just for you but for your whole family. If you can do it by adding herbs or other healthy veggies, go right ahead. Maybe you want peppers in everything or you want to add potatoes. Maybe you favor cumin in slaw and that works for you. Or paprika. And if that includes adding marshmallows and peanuts to slaw—yes, I really do that—to get kids to eat it, that's fine; any way you can get cabbage down their little throats is okay by me.

I'm not saying put a cup of blue cheese dressing on a stalk of broccoli. Use a minimalist approach: just enough and no more. The focus is on eating the right types of vegetables and fruit, but if I'm eating slaw or broccoli every day, I want to vary the flavor and the texture. That may mean using a little sugar or some fat as in mayonnaise. Experiment with the recipes to vary the flavor and make them fit your taste. The goal is to eat the right foods—enhancing the flavor is a plus.

Basic Cabbage Soup

6 cloves garlic
1 – 2 large Vidalia or sweet onions, sliced
2 tablespoons extra-virgin olive oil
4 16-ounce cans vegetarian broth or two 32-ounce boxes
4 cups water
1 large head cabbage, chopped fine
1 large leek, washed and thinly sliced
2 teaspoons chopped fresh sage, one teaspoon dried
    sage, or ¾ teaspoon ground sage
2 teaspoons sea salt (or salt to taste)
1 teaspoon Tabasco sauce or other hot sauce (optional)
Pepper to taste
2 tablespoons apple cider vinegar (optional)

In a large stock pot, slowly sauté garlic and onions in olive oil until translucent, being careful not to let them burn. Add broth, water, cabbage, leek, spices, and salt. Bring to a boil. Reduce heat and simmer for 30 – 60 minutes. Experiment with various spices to vary the flavor. If you prefer a more tart taste, add the apple cider vinegar.

The nice thing about this soup is that it can last for days.

Basic Detox Coleslaw

This is a recipe I discovered while watching a grilling show. It was such a great approach instead of the typical green cabbage with many more phytonutrients, and the dressing is delicious.

Dressing (Double Batch)
¼ cup lemon juice
¼ cup orange juice
2 tablespoons clover honey
2 tablespoons Dijon mustard
¼ cup fresh basil leaves, chopped
½ cup canola oil
Seasonings such as salt and pepper to taste

Slaw
2 cups thinly sliced Napa cabbage
2 cups thinly sliced red cabbage
1 large carrot, peeled and grated very coarsely

Put the lemon juice, orange juice, honey, mustard, basil and some salt and pepper in a blender and blend until smooth.

Combine the Napa cabbage, red cabbage, and carrot in a large bowl; add not quite half the dressing and toss to coat. Season with salt and pepper, and add more dressing if needed.

Want a sweeter taste or more crunch when you move on to daily detox? Add dried cherries, craisins, walnuts, or sliced almonds for a change of pace. You could even add a bit of fruit or other vegetables, add herbs, or vary the spices from time to time. Because the more you like the slaw, the easier it is to eat, and that's the goal.

Creamy Coleslaw

1 tablespoons sugar
1 tablespoons apple cider vinegar
¼ cup salad dressing such as Miracle Whip
½ cup mayonnaise
Salt and pepper to taste

4 cups of chopped cabbage, any type or a mixture
1 carrot, peeled and grated

Blend the dressing ingredients together. Pour over the cabbage and carrots and mix thoroughly.

I know what you're thinking: what kind of detox program uses that much fat? You can modify it if you want, but this coleslaw can become a staple of your daily detox, so make it the way you like best. More ways to reduce calories:

Use stevia or other artificial sweetener instead of sugar
Use light salad dressing
Use light mayonnaise

This is my recipe, and I use real sugar and real mayonnaise. But they're not the show—the cabbage is. I want to satisfy my taste buds. Calories don't matter as much when your goal is to detox, but go low fat and low sugar if you want to.

Kid-Friendly Version
1 small can pineapple tidbits (about 1 cup)
1 cup miniature marshmallows
¾ cup cocktail or dry-roasted salted peanuts

Adding these to the creamy coleslaw makes it more appealing to young palates, and adults like the salty-sweet taste as well. It doesn't keep well, so add these as you go.

Cabbage Stew

In this recipe, there are more vegetables and the vegetables are cut more coarsely to give the impression of a more substantial food than soup.

4 cloves garlic, chopped fine
3 – 4 medium onions, chopped coarsely or sliced
2 tablespoons extra-virgin olive oil
4 16-ounce cans vegetarian broth or two 32-ounce boxes
4 cups water
1 large head of cabbage, chopped coarsely
2 large carrots, sliced
12 – 18 Brussels sprouts, cut in half
1 red pepper chopped
2 tablespoons chopped fresh oregano or 1 tablespoon dried
  oregano
2 teaspoons sea salt (or salt to taste)
Pepper to taste

In a large stock pot, slowly sauté garlic and onions in olive oil until translucent, being careful not to let them burn.

Add broth, water, cabbage, carrots, Brussels sprouts, red pepper, spices, and salt. Bring to a boil. Reduce heat and simmer for 30 – 60 minutes or until vegetables are tender.

"I Can't Cook" Detox Cabbage Soup

No experience necessary—your five-year-old could make this soup. Simply open jars and bags, empty the contents into a pan, and heat. It can't get much easier than this!

2 16-ounce bags of coleslaw mix from the produce section at your grocery
4 16-ounce cans of vegetarian broth or two 32-ounce boxes
4 cups water
1 10-ounce bag of frozen diced onions
2 tablespoons chopped garlic from a jar, also usually in the produce section
1 small bag petite-cut carrots
2 teaspoons sea salt (or salt to taste)
1 teaspoon Tabasco sauce or other hot sauce (optional)
Pepper to taste

Combine all ingredients in a large stock pot. Bring to a boil, then reduce heat and simmer over low heat until vegetables are tender, stirring occasionally. Check seasonings and add more sea salt and/or Tabasco to taste.

Cauliflower & Broccoli Detox Soup

If you want the texture and look of a creamy soup, try this recipe. To maintain color and flavor, cook the broccoli only until it's warm.

4 cloves garlic, chopped fine
3 – 4 medium onions, chopped fine
2 tablespoons extra-virgin olive oil
2 cups water
1 12-ounce bag frozen cauliflower flowerets
3 16-ounce cans vegetarian broth
1 10-ounce box frozen collard greens (optional)
1 teaspoon ground ginger
1 teaspoon ground cumin or curry powder
2 teaspoons sea salt (or salt to taste)
1 12-ounce bag frozen broccoli flowerets
Pepper to taste

In a large stock pot, slowly sauté garlic and onions in olive oil until translucent, being careful not to let them burn.

Add water and cauliflower; cook until the cauliflower is tender, then pour it into a food processor and blend or if you use a stick blender, blend in pot until smooth.

Return it to the pot, and add the broth, collard greens, spices, and salt. Bring to a boil again. Reduce heat, and add broccoli flowerets. Cook until broccoli is hot and check seasonings; remove from heat to keep broccoli greener.

Broccoli-Cauliflower Detox Salad

Dressing (Double Batch)
1 tablespoons sugar
1 tablespoons apple cider vinegar
¼ cup salad dressing such as Miracle Whip
½ cup mayonnaise (both low fat if you prefer)
Salt and pepper to taste

Salad
1 bunch broccoli
½ head cauliflower
2 green onions
2 tablespoons sunflower seeds

Blend the dressing ingredients together (this is the same dressing as the Creamy Coleslaw and makes a double batch; save half for coleslaw tomorrow). Cut veggies into bite-size pieces and mix together with half the dressing just before serving.

To liven up this salad a bit when you reach daily detox, try this variation, based on my mother-in-law's family-favorite recipe. Add these ingredients to the dressing, which is better when prepared a day ahead to allow the flavors to blend:

¼ cup grated Parmesan cheese
2 tablespoons bacon or turkey bacon pieces (or 2 bacon strips crumbled)
½ teaspoon Mrs. Dash or other seasoning blend

Bacon? Yes—the important point is that you're getting the cruciferous vegetables your body needs to detox; a little bit of bacon and cheese won't negate that.

Squash Detox Soup

Let's face it: you're getting a little weary of green vegetables. Here's a detox soup of a different color as well as a slightly different flavor. One of the less-familiar ingredients is daikon, a white Chinese radish that has great flavor.

4 cloves garlic, chopped fine
3 – 4 medium onions, chopped fine
2 tablespoons extra-virgin olive oil
2 cups water
1 large daikon (Chinese radish), chopped into 1-inch cubes
3 16-ounce cans vegetarian broth
2 16-ounce cans cooked squash* or fresh squash
  or pumpkin, peeled and cut into cubes
1 teaspoon ground ginger
1 teaspoon ground nutmeg
2 teaspoons sea salt (or salt to taste) and pepper to taste

In a large stock pot, slowly sauté garlic and onions in olive oil until translucent, being careful not to let them burn. Add water, squash (if you used fresh), and daikon; cook until the daikon is tender. Place in a food processor and blend.

Return to pot and add the broth, squash (if you used canned), spices, and salt. Bring to a boil again and remove from heat.

For a sweeter taste, add agave nectar or stevia a little at a time until the taste is slightly sweet and slightly nutty.

*If you can't find cooked squash in a can, you can substitute an orange squash such as acorn squash you cook yourself to get about four cups (just pierce it several times with a fork and microwave until it softens); you also can use sweet potatoes or pumpkin from a can or prepare them yourself.

Mushroom Detox Soup

The type of mushrooms used will dictate the color, from golden brown to dark brown.

2 pounds mushrooms, chopped, any type
3 tablespoons extra-virgin olive oil
2 large celery stalks, chopped
4 large garlic cloves, chopped
4 shallots, thinly sliced
2 medium leeks, chopped
4 16-ounce cans vegetarian broth or two 32-ounce boxes
2 bay leaves
3 sprigs fresh thyme or 1 teaspoon dried thyme
Salt and pepper to taste

In a large stock pot, heat the olive oil on high heat until the oil starts lightly smoking. Add mushrooms and stir constantly until the mushrooms are golden brown on the edges, about five minutes. Add celery, garlic, shallots, and leeks. Stir constantly until the shallots are translucent, being careful not to burn the vegetables.

Add the vegetarian broth slowly because the hot pan will cause the broth to spatter. Add bay leaves, thyme, and salt; bring to a boil for 30 minutes. Remove the bay leaves and sprigs of thyme.

Creamy Mushroom Detox Soup

For a a creamy soup without butter or cream, prepare as above, reserving ½ pound of mushrooms. After boiling, remove from heat and let cool for 15 – 30 minutes. Pour soup into a blender or food processor and blend until smooth. Sauté the remaining ½ pound of mushrooms in one tablespoon olive oil until browned. Reduce heat, add soup, and reheat.

Berry Combo

No matter which fruits you use, this is a phytonutrient goldmine!

These are the most important berries, and you should always use at least one of them. If you prefer citrus, pineapple, or other fruits, go for it, but always start with these:

Black raspberries	Red grapes
Blueberries	Red raspberries
Dark cherries	Strawberries

Using fresh or frozen fruit (thawed or semi-thawed for eating), mix together any proportions of the fruits listed above to equal one cup. Drizzle with one teaspoon of agave nectar, stevia, or honey. Experiment with herbs: basil and mint are most common, but add cilantro if that's how you roll. Stir thoroughly and eat.

When you move on to the daily detox, adding a squirt of whipped cream or a scoop of low-fat ice cream makes this even more of a treat. Once again, the point is to continue getting the phytonutrients, and if eating the right foods is enjoyable as well, even better.

Protein Drink

Use any kind of frozen juice, even mixes such as piña colada or fuzzy navel.

½ cup water
¼ cup crushed ice
¼ cup frozen fruit-juice concentrate
1 tablespoon vegetarian protein powder, either rice or soy
2 teaspoons soluble fiber such as guar gum or inulin fiber

Place ingredients in blender and mix for 60 seconds or until smooth.

If you like the taste of vegetable juice, use that for the basis of your drink instead of fruit; eliminate the water and possibly the ice, depending on taste. For a different flavor, add any hot sauce or spices you like.

Chunky Protein Drink

If the berries are tart, add up to two teaspoons agave nectar, stevia, or honey.

½ cup water
¼ cup crushed ice (optional if berries are frozen)
½ cup fresh or frozen berries of your choice
1 tablespoon vegetarian protein powder, either rice or soy
2 teaspoons soluble fiber such as guar gum or inulin fiber

Place water, protein powder, and fiber, plus ice and sweetener if used, in blender and mix until smooth. Add berries and pulse or mix briefly until ingredients are mixed but berries are still chunky. Experiment with herbs such as basil and mint to vary the flavor.